Folk Medicine

Folk Medicine

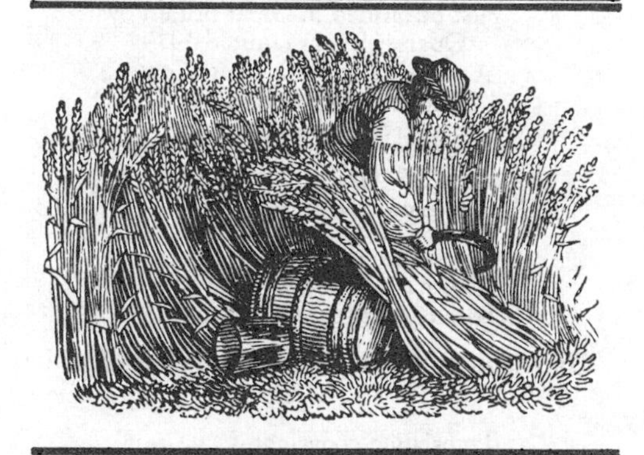

JACQUES VEISSID

Translated from the French by
NADIA LEGRAND

QUARTET BOOKS
LONDON · MELBOURNE · NEW YORK

First published in Great Britain by
Quartet Books Limited 1979
A member of the Namara Group
27 Goodge Street, London W1P 1FD

Published by arrangement with
The K.S. Giniger Company Inc.,
235 Park Avenue South, New York City, 10003

First published under the title
Traité de Médecine Populaire by
Société Parisienne d'Édition 1973

ISBN 0 7043 3298 1

Designed by Mike Jarvis

Typeset by Clerkenwell Graphics

Printed and bound in Great Britain
by Hazell, Watson and Viney Ltd.
Aylesbury, Bucks.

Contents

Part 2

Introduction

For some time interest has been growing in popular or folk medicine and 'natural' remedies prepared from herbs as alternatives to pharmaceutical products.

This book has been assembled from the popular medicine procedures published by the *Almanach Vermot* which is read widely throughout the French countryside. The *Almanach* has been ideally suited for over a century to gather at source a very full documentation of folk remedies, including those that were for long believed to owe their effect to the 'magic' properties of which so much was made of by the 'healers'.

Until the last century most peasants lived in isolation and to fetch a doctor often meant a long and often difficult journey. Each family, therefore, had to deal at home with injuries and sickness and methods of treatment were handed down from generation to generation much as recipes and kitchen lore were. Some passed from one 'healer' to another. Others, again, were learned by nuns, doctors and health officers from those they visited in country districts.

Popular medicine may therefore be called the medicine of first aid or the medicine of necessity and this definition sets the limits of what it can do. The methods are often efficacious but in the main should be regarded as temporary measures and sometimes desperate remedies. For example, if a sick person has a sudden and dramatic rise in body temperature a popular treatment may be used to bring the fever down but it would be dangerous to believe that the patient is cured. What has been achieved is a successful treatment of the most urgent problem, carried out as a safety measure until the doctor arrives.

At the same time it is foolish to trust blindly in herbal

remedies as practised in the country. Pharmaceutical science has identified the active properties of plants and has used them in a way that will produce quicker results than by using the plants themselves. But more or less regular use of certain herbs can be beneficial to general health.

In certain afflictions which are not serious, such as colds, sore throats, some skin diseases, corns, warts, minor ulcers, slight burns and sprains, it may be possible to provide treatment by folk methods which *might* produce better results than those achieved by orthodox medicine.

In short, folk medicine can be of great use but it should not be forgotten that it is a branch of medicine that has remained static since the last century. It would therefore be unreasonable and unrealistic to expect it to possess greater over-all efficacy than scientific medicine which is a 'living' science that moves forward constantly.

JACQUES VEISSID

Foreword

BY THE TRANSLATOR TO THE ENGLISH EDITION

As Jacques Veissid makes clear in his introduction, the remedies described in this book have been gathered from many rural sources in provincial France. For the most part they were transmitted through oral tradition and the unsophisticated directness of peasant speech and vocabulary is evident throughout the French original. I have retained this simplicity and sometimes its old-fashioned turns of phrase as well. References to such outmoded articles as a *seau hygiénique* – like the slop pails of our rustic ancestors, or the vague generalizations like 'back ache' and 'stitch' and the setting out of cures for medieval afflictions such as the King's Evil have been set down faithfully in the English even though they may merely raise a smile in whichever language they appear.

Certain fundamental differences did present themselves for which no ready English equivalents can be found. Medicinal alcohol of varying proof or even *eau de vie* are not as ready to hand as they are in France. Neither are cauldrons, coffee-bowls, orange and olive trees and the Mediterranean herbs that grow as weeds in many parts of France but must be taken from the herbalist's jar here. And it must be remembered that a coffeespoon is equivalent to a *small* teaspoon.

The Latin names of plants are not given in the French edition but I have added them to the list of preparations in the English edition in the interests of accuracy and safety. Only by checking the common names against the botanical names can one be sure of what one is doing. Common names vary from county to county, sometimes from village to village. The English bluebell is a wild hyacinth in Scotland and the Scottish bluebell is a harebell in England and the plants belong to different families anyway. When you see that the name of a plant includes *'officinalis'* you can be sure that it was used medicinally from the Latin *officina*, originally 'workshop' and then a 'herb-store' and 'drug-shop'. There is a note relative to this in the introduction to Part 2: The Preparations.

NADIA LEGRAND

How to use this book

The book is divided into two parts:

(1) The first part lists illnesses and conditions and the popular medicine methods suggested for dealing with them. They are not arranged alphabetically but by groups classified by the parts or functions of the body dealt with under each heading, e.g. circulation, digestion, the skeleton, etc. In this way the reader who does not know the name of the illness that confronts him or cannot distinguish, for instance, between tonsilitis, laryngitis and pharyngitis, can find the remedy suggested by looking under the appropriate anatomical or symptomatic heading, in this case under sore throat in the part dealing with the Respiratory System. Having found the right heading he will find what treatment to give and sometimes be referred to the second part of the book for instructions in the preparation of the infusion, decoction, tincture, etc. that is required.

(2) The second part gives the recipes for the principal preparations used in popular medicine. Each has a number and it is under that number that they are referred to in the first part, thus making them easy to find.

In addition to finding there the instructions for preparing what is needed, the reader will find, under the names of plants used in these treatments, which specific illnesses are treated by each one.

Part One

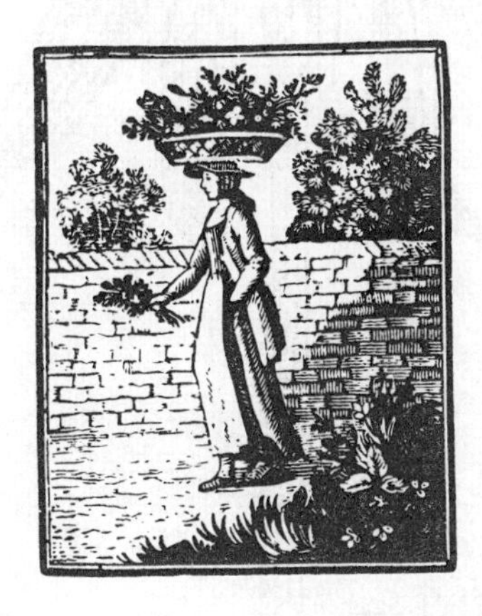

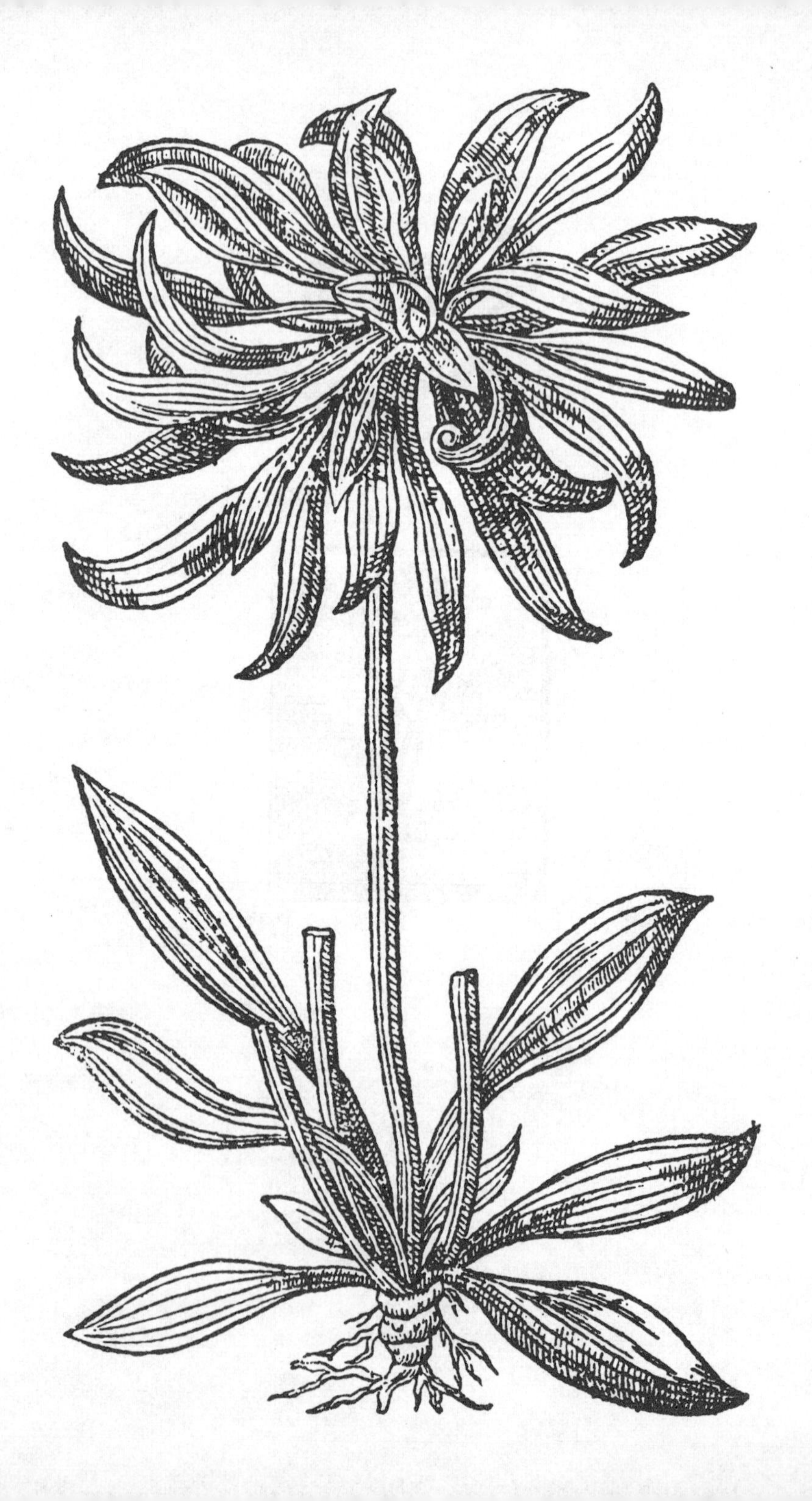

Minor Injuries and Mild Mishaps

ABSCESSES · ANTHRAX · INJURIES · BURNS · CONTUSIONS
HEAT STROKE · CUTS · CRACKED SKIN
EXPULSION OF FOREIGN BODIES · CARBUNCLES · HICCUPS
ANIMAL BITES · INFLAMMATION · VARIOUS INSECT BITES
WASP AND BEE STINGS · SPIDER BITES · MOSQUITO BITES
NETTLE STINGS · WARTS

ABSCESSES

Abscesses are formed by a collection of pus, namely an accumulation under the skin of dead white cells and bacteria. Pain, often severe, is caused by the pressure of pus in the flesh. To 'ripen the abscess', a remedy suggested by popular medicine, the pus is drawn into one spot and the skin there is softened in such a way that the pustular matter can come out.

When the abscess breaks there is immediate relief. It must be remembered, however, that an abscess is the result of infection and therefore the ailment is not necessarily terminated after the abscess has been brought to a head.

Diet for people prone to abscesses

Some people are more subject to abscesses than others. This is due to poor general health which may be improved, according to popular tradition, by a diet of fresh vegetables and fresh fruit juices. This diet should be adhered to for one week in each month and during that time a coffeespoonful of brewer's yeast should be taken with the midday and evening meals.

Dried fig method

Cook a large dried fig in milk until soft. Cut the fig in half and apply the inner surface to the abscess, covering it with a piece of flannel held in place by a strip of crêpe bandage.

The fig must be used when very hot but taking care that it does not scald. Repeat the treatment with another fig every three hours until the abscess has been brought to a head.

Egg Method

Beat a fresh egg as though for an omelette and while stirring add three tablespoonfuls of best white flour. Cook the preparation in a *bain marie* (double saucepan) until a thick paste has been obtained. Wrap in a piece of gauze and apply to the abscess and fix in place with a crêpe bandage. Repeat the treatment every three hours.

Honey ointment method

Mix equal amounts of honey, butter, lard and salt. Start by mixing the butter with the honey, then beat in the lard and finally add the salt.

Apply a generous quantity of this ointment to the abscess and cover with a piece of gauze and a crêpe bandage.

Sundry methods

Carrot: grate coarsely a raw carrot and apply the pulp to the abscess. Cover with a gauze dressing and crêpe bandage. Repeat the treatment every two hours.

Bread: remove the crust from several slices of bread and soak the slices for a quarter of an hour in tepid milk. Strain off a liquid and apply the soggy bread as a poultice to the abscess. Cover with gauze and crêpe bandage. Repeat the treatment every two or three hours.

Flour: mix equal quantities of honey and flour. Apply to the abscess the preparation wrapped in gauze and covered with the crêpe bandage or sticking plaster. Repeat every two or three hours.

Walnut: chew two or three walnuts until they are soaked with saliva and then apply this in the form of a poultice to the abscess. Cover with gauze held in place by sticking plaster and renew the treatment every four hours.

ANTHRAX

A cabbage leaf dressing (preparation No. 55) is considered to be very effective in the treatment of anthrax. The dressing should be renewed every four hours. Should the pain become unbearable, however, a dressing should be applied at more frequent intervals. It should be noted that all treatments for abscesses are also applicable in cases of anthrax.

INJURIES

Under the heading of injuries we are only considering sores, grazes and such superficial scratches as may reasonably be considered not to be serious. Obviously, in the case of a serious lesion, a doctor should be called as soon as possible.

First-aid measure

If there is nothing to hand with which to disinfect a wound and stop the bleeding the following may be used as palliative methods.

Oil and wine: pour into a bottle a glass of olive oil and an equal amount of red wine. Shake well so as to produce an emulsion and bathe the injury with the liquid.

Walnut: ask the patient to chew two or three walnuts or, if he is unable to do so, chew them yourself and when the nuts have been reduced to a paste and well soaked with saliva apply the mixture to the injury.

Sugar: crush to a fine powder with a rolling pin or bottle some lumps of sugar and then sprinkle it on the wound.

Nettles: pound some stinging nettle leaves in a mortar or chop them finely with a knife. Apply to the wound.

Geranium: crush lightly with a rolling pin or bottle some geranium leaves and apply them to the injury.

Lady's mantle: soak fresh lady's mantle leaves in water for a short while and then apply the undersides of the leaves to the wound.

Ash twig method: there is some doubt as to the efficacy of the following treatment but it has long been renowned in many regions of France and is therefore listed here. Cut an undamaged and healthy ash twig in spring and preferably at the time of the first new moon following 21 March. Cut each end of the twig cleanly and seal thoroughly with wax to prevent the sap from evaporating. According to popular tradition a brief contact between the twig and the injury will hasten the process of healing. *(Translator's note:* it should, however, not be forgotten that an open wound is susceptible to infection; contact with a non-sterile object will automatically introduce bacteria into the wound field, some of which may be pathogenic, i.e. capable of producing infection.)

Sundry treatments

Mugwort: add to a litre of cold water three tablespoonfuls of mugwort leaves. Place in a saucepan and bring gently to the boil and allow to infuse for half an hour. Strain through fine muslin and add two tablespoonfuls of rock salt. Soak compresses with this liquid and place them on the wound, renewing the treatment twice daily. *(Translator's note:* wound healing is favoured by drying; application of a watery liquid could lead to ideal conditions for bacterial multiplication and sustain infection.)

Lily: macerate for six hours lily petals in *eau de vie* 45°. Apply the petals to the wound, cover with gauze and hold in place with a bandage. *(Translator's note:* Madonna lily petals should be used).

Tansy: put into a saucepan ten tablespoonfuls of tansy flowers to a litre of cold water. Bring slowly to the boil, simmer for a quarter of an hour and strain. Bathe the wound twice a day with this decoction which is said to be particularly effective in the case of infected sores.

Marigold: chop coarsely some marigold flowers. Wrap them in a piece of gauze fixed in place over the wound by a bandage.

Garlic or onion: take the outer skin of a clove of garlic or an onion and apply the inside surface to the wound. This treatment is particularly helpful in dealing with scratches.

Veronica: a sore may be disinfected by bathing it with a decoction of veronica (preparation No. 161).

Lavender: lavender infusions (preparation No. 94) can be used on compresses and are considered to be very efficacious in wound repair. They should be renewed every two hours.

Shepherd's purse: apply to the wound a gauze soaked with shepherd's purse wine (preparation No. 36a) and kept in place by a bandage. Shepherd's purse wine is considered to be very useful in the healing of bed sores; in this case, however, the compress should be applied for about ten minutes only.
St John's wort: bathe wounds in oil of St John's wort (preparation No. 109) several times a day.
Sage: Apply compresses soaked with an infusion of sage (preparation No. 145) and secure them in place on the wound with a bandage. This method is reputed to be particularly effective when the wound is suppurating.

BURNS

Popular medicine offers in the case of burns an abundance of treatments, most of which are very efficacious and bring almost instant relief. However, one should be careful to treat in this way only burns that are superficial and of small extent. Any serious burn requires urgent medical attention.

Potato dressing

This method brings swift relief provided it is instituted promptly after the injury. Cut a raw potato in half. Grate it and apply the pulp to the burn. Fifteen minutes' application is often enough to relieve the pain completely and initiate rapid wound repair. However, to be on the safe side, grate another potato and wrap it in a gauze to have it ready to apply should a second poultice be needed. Never use the potato skin – only the pulp should be grated.

White of egg

Beat the white of an egg until stiff and apply immediately to the burn. For greater effect, however, add to the white of egg three tablespoonfuls of olive oil whisked with a fork as for an omelette. Apply several times and at brief intervals more of the preparation without removing the preceding layers.

Yolk of egg

Mix the yolk of an egg with an equal volume of softened butter until the resultant ointment can be applied to the burn.

Whole egg

Beat in a bowl an egg while adding to it olive oil as for mayonnaise until a creamy consistency is obtained. Apply to the burn, repeating at short intervals.

Oil of box leaves

This medication must be prepared in advance and stored for use when needed.

Pound in a mortar five tablespoonfuls of fresh boxwood leaves. Place the ground leaves in a bottle together with half a litre of olive oil. Allow the preparation to macerate for a week, shaking the bottle twice a day. Filter it at the end of the week. Apply to the burn either by dabbing it on with cotton wool or by a soft paintbrush.

Sundry methods

Sodium bicarbonate: moisten bicarbonate of soda with a few drops of vinegar. Apply the preparation to the burn.
Carrots: peel and finely grate some carrots. Apply the pulp to the burn and hold in place with a gauze compress.
Cabbage: pound some cabbage leaves with a pestle and apply to the burn.
Pumpkin: apply the flesh of crushed pumpkin to the burn and fix it in place with a strip of gauze. Crushed vegetable marrow or gourd flesh may be used in the same way.
Comfrey: grate a fresh root of comfrey. Apply to the burn and hold in place with gauze.
Glycerine: by means of cotton wool or a cloth well soaked with glycerine cover the whole burn area, making sure that the contiguous tissues are also covered.
Ivy: dip some ivy leaves in boiling water. Crush them and bring them to the boil again, adding several spoonfuls of *eau de vie* to the water. Wrap the preparation in gauze and apply to the burn.

Melon: mash the flesh of a melon and apply it to the burn.
Honey: apply to the burn gauze compresses previously soaked with honey. Cover with a bandage.
St John's wort: gently dab the burn with a wad of cotton wool soaked with St John's wort oil (preparation No. 109). Apply several times at intervals of fifteen minutes.
Onion: slice thinly an onion, sprinkle with salt, mash with a fork and apply to the burn. Cover with a gauze compress.
Spinach: brown some spinach in olive oil. When cooled apply to the burn.
Salt: if nothing else is available bathe the burns with water containing 40 g of salt to the litre.
Marigold: chop finely fresh marigold flowers and wrap them in a strip of gauze. Apply to the burn.

CONTUSIONS

The following measures may be applied to the various injuries resulting from blows or falls, etc. where the skin is not broken, and regardless whether or not bumps or bruises are visible.

Blows to the head

Cut into small pieces some bread from which the crust has been removed. Cook in a small amount of red wine until a fairly thick and smooth paste is obtained. Remove the saucepan from the heat source and add one tablespoonful of olive oil. Mix thoroughly. Wrap the preparation in a thin cloth or a piece of gauze and apply as hot as is bearable to the injury. Repeat when the poultice has cooled. *(Translators note:* Any blow to the head that results in a period of unconsciousness, however brief and even if it is followed by a period of apparent recovery, should be treated as a medical emergency and be referred instantly to the nearest hospital accident and emergency department.)

Bruised fingers

Pound in a mortar three tablespoonfuls of chopped parsley with one tablespoonful of salt. Moisten with a spoonful of *eau de vie* or olive oil. Rub the liquid on the bruises and apply it to the whole surface of injured fingers with the chopped parsley, holding it in place with gauze and a bandage. (*Translator's note:* it should not be forgotten that persistent pain and inflammation may suggest fracture).

Various treatments for all manner of contusions

Agrimony: put in a saucepan five tablespoonfuls of agrimony leaves, pour on it half a litre of boiling water. Cook for a quarter of an hour and allow to infuse for a further five minutes. Strain and soak a compress with the decoction which is then applied to the injury. When the compress has cooled renew the treatment.
Parsley: apply a poultice of chopped parsley held in place by a bandage.
White of egg: beat the white of an egg until it is stiff. Spread on a fine cloth and apply to the bruises.
Black bryony: in some parts of France this plant is called the 'herb of the beaten woman'. Pound very carefully fresh leaves until the paste obtained can be applied to the bruises.
Crane's bill: pound in a mortar fresh leaves of crane's bill. Apply the ground leaves to the injury.
Arnica: prepare the following decoction of arnica. Put in a saucepan three tablespoonfuls of arnica flowers to half a litre of cold water. (If the plant is not in bloom use the leaves instead.) Bring slowly to the boil and boil for ten minutes, strain and place in a small receptable packed around with ice. When the decoction is thoroughly chilled, soak a compress with it. Apply to the injury and repeat with another compress when the first one has become tepid.

HEAT STROKE

According to popular tradition when somebody has lost consciousness as a result of heat stroke blood should be drawn from the lobe of the ear by making a small incision.

CUTS

Nettle poultice

Nettles have long been used to stop bleeding from minor cuts.

Start by cleaning the wound with either peroxide of hydrogen, salt water or by lemon juice mixed with twice its volume of water. Gather fresh roots of stinging nettles. Wash and dry them carefully. Crush finely and apply a substantial amount to the cut, holding in place with a dressing.

Alternative methods

Geranium: apply to the cut some crushed geranium leaves. Hold in place with a dressing.
Cabbage: roll into a ball between the hands a cabbage leaf. Flatten the leaf and apply it to the wound.

CRACKED SKIN

Oak bark lotion

Bathing the hands with oak bark lotion is considered very effective in the treatment of cracked skin. Prepare a decoction as follows: place in a saucepan six tablespoonfuls of chips of oak bark to one litre of water. Bring slowly to the boil, keep it on the boil for half an hour and then strain. Soak the hands in this liquid for fifteen minutes three times a day. The preparation should be warmed up again whenever it is needed.

Likewise the following decoction can also be helpful: put in a saucepan five tablespoonfuls of chopped oak bark, five of chopped walnut bark. Add five tablespoonfuls of agrimony leaves and two tablespoonfuls of lavender flowers. Add a litre of water. Bring slowly to the boil, boil for a quarter of an hour and strain. Soak the hands in this decoction for ten minutes three times daily.

Sundry methods

Cabbage: apply to the cracked skin pieces of cabbage leaves

which have previously been dipped in olive oil.
Candle wax: hold a lighted candle at an angle above the cracked skin. Allow the wax to drip on to the cracks and allow it to remain in place until it comes off of its own accord. Repeat the treatment three times a day.
Olive oil: massage the cracked skin with a mixture of equal parts of olive oil and glycerine.

EXPLUSION OF FOREIGN BODIES

Potato method

This treatment is used when the patient has swallowed a small foreign body such as a piece of glass or a chip of enamel which might injure the stomach or bowels. Prepare a stiff mixture of mashed potatoes and get the patient to eat it until there is a sensation of fullness in the stomach. No liquid should be drunk for at least two hours.

Leek method

Cook a leek in boiling water or in a steamer. It should then be chewed only enough to allow it to be swallowed as whole as possible without difficulty.

CARBUNCLES

All the methods described above for the treatment of abscesses and anthrax can also be used for carbuncles. However, the following are specific treatments.

Leek method

Place the white part of three leeks in a saucepan and barely cover them with water, adding six lumps of sugar. Cook very slowly until the water has evaporated. Crush the leeks until they are completely reduced to a paste. Wrap in gauze and apply the poultice to the carbuncle, keeping it in place with a crêpe bandage or sticking plaster.

Burdock method

Boil fresh leaves and roots of burdock in a small quantity of water for ten minutes. Strain, crush the leaves and roots and apply the preparation to the carbuncle. Cover with a piece of gauze held in place by a bandage or plaster. Repeat the treatment after twelve hours.

Mullein method

Gather fresh leaves of mullein. Boil them in milk for five minutes and apply them as hot as possible to the carbuncle. Cover with a piece of gauze held in place appropriately. Renew the poultice after twelve hours.

Sundry methods

Bean flour: mix bean flour with a small quantity of water to form a thick paste which is then wrapped in a piece of gauze and applied as a poultice to the carbuncle. Renew every six hours.
Sorrel: brown a few leaves of sorrel in butter. When cooked, crush the leaves gently with a fork. Wrap the leaves in a piece of gauze and apply to the carbuncle, holding the poultice in place with sticking plaster or a bandage. Renew the treatment twice a day.
Bindweed: shred by hand some bindweed leaves. Use a generous amount of the torn leaves and apply immediately to the carbuncle. The gauze used to cover it should be held by a crêpe bandage or other suitable means. Renew the treatment after six hours.

HICCUPS

Vinegar method

To swallow straight down a coffeespoonful of vinegar is one of the most effective remedies for hiccups. Another way is to soak a lump of sugar with vinegar and allow it to dissolve on the tongue.

Hot water method

Fill a wash basin with water as hot as it can be borne and soak the hands in it for ten minutes.

Other methods

Pepper: chew slowly three peppercorns.
Wood calamint: drink two cupfuls of calamint infusion (preparation No. 42) at ten-minute intervals.
Mint: drink a hot infusion of mint (preparation No. 106) and, if needed, another one fifteen minutes later.
Orange leaves: drink a cupful of hot infusion of orange tree leaves (preparation No. 119).

ANIMAL BITES

Always treat an animal bite as a potentially serious injury which must be seen quickly by a doctor. For that reason the following methods should only be considered as first-aid measures.

Measures to guard against adder bites

According to popular tradition the smell of musk is abhorrent to reptiles and therefore smearing the legs with musk would have the effect of repelling them.

Adder bites

Make an incision at the point where the adder's fangs have pierced the flesh and suck the wound, remembering to spit out the blood and rinse the mouth. It is said that the action of the venom can be delayed by drinking a glass of olive oil. Obviously this is only a supplementary first-aid measure and one must always take the patient as swiftly as possible to the nearest doctor.

Other animal bites

The following methods can be used in the treatment of bites by dogs, cats and small wild animals. Large animal bites such as those inflicted by a horse or cow produce too deep lesions to be treated satisfactorily at home and a doctor should be consulted at once.

Onion method

Popular medicine considers onion as being the specific treatment for animal bites. Crush thoroughly an onion, sprinkling it frequently with salt. Spread the preparation over the bite, cover with a gauze compress and maintain in place with a dressing until the next day when Samaritan balm (preparation No. 117) is applied.

Other methods

French beans: pound as fine as possible some French bean pods or leaves. Apply them to the bite and cover with a gauze compress secured by a dressing.
Mint: proceed as above, substituting mint leaves.
Nettles: pound in a mortar some stinging nettle leaves, sprinkling them frequently with salt. Spread the preparation on the bite and cover with a dressing. If a pestle and mortar are not available chop finely the nettle leaves, sprinkling them with salt.

PHLEGMON or INFLAMMATION

All the treatments applicable to abscesses, carbuncles and anthrax are equally effective in the case of inflammation or, to use the old term, phlegmon. Furthermore the following method may be considered as the specific. Take a lily bulb and cook it in milk. When soft it should be mashed with a fork and then wrapped in a piece of gauze and applied to the inflammation. Hold it in place with a crêpe bandage or other appropriate dressing. Renew after twelve hours.

VARIOUS INSECT BITES

These procedures may be used in the treatment of insect bites even when it is not known which insect has inflicted them.

Blackcurrent leaves

Rub freshly crushed blackcurrant leaves on the bite.

Cabbage leaf

Rub the bite with a fresh cabbage leaf which has been crumpled in the hand. Following this, apply a piece of the leaf to the sting and fix it in place with sticking plaster.

Leek

Cut through the white part of a leek and rub the bite with the cut surface.

Parsley

Chop some parsley, apply to the bite and cover with a small gauze compress held in place with a sticking plaster.

Thyme

Rub fresh thyme on the bite.

Horseradish

Chop some horseradish root and apply it to the bite, covering with gauze held in place with sticking plaster.

WASP AND BEE STINGS

When you realize that you are in the process of being stung by a bee or wasp do not attempt to squash the insect *in situ*. If the sting has been left in the skin it should be removed with a needle that has previously been sterilized in a flame. Try to get the wound to bleed. One may then employ one of the undermentioned procedures. (*Translator's note:* Wasp and bee stings may elicit in certain individuals a reaction which may be so severe as sometimes to prove fatal. It follows that any victim manifesting signs throughout the whole body, i.e. difficulty in breathing, fainting, nausea and undue flushing should be referred as an acute medical urgency to a doctor. Such a reaction is, however, very rare.)

Bites in the mouth

One should first examine a fruit before biting into it to make sure that it does not shelter a wasp. A bite inside the throat and mouth can be most dangerous and a doctor should be called at once. Meanwhile gargle with cold water.

Preventive method

According to popular belief protection against bee and wasp stings is set up if the exposed parts of the body are rubbed with walnut leaves or tomato leaves that have been previously crumpled.

Garlic

Cut in two a peeled clove of garlic and rub the sting with the cut surface.

Tincture of iodine

Dab the sting with a wad of cotton wool damped with tincture of iodine.

Salt water

Apply to the sting a compress soaked with cold and heavily salted water.

Onion

Rub the sting with an onion cut in half; then place a slice of onion on the sting and strap it in place with sticking plaster.

Vinegar

Dissolve salt to saturation point in a little vinegar. Apply to the sting a compress soaked in the liquid.

SPIDER BITES

Garlic

First wash the bite with a piece of cotton wool dipped in hot vinegar then apply some crushed garlic and hold in place with a small dressing.

Leek

Chop finely a piece of leek. Crush it in a mortar, mixing it with a little honey. Apply this to the bite and cover with a gauze compress.

MOSQUITO BITES

Parsley

Rub the bite with crumpled parsley.

Leek

Chop finely a small piece of leek. Apply it to the bite and hold in place with a piece of gauze.

Vinegar and lemon juice

Mix a coffeespoonful of vinegar with an equal quantity of lemon juice. Dab the sting with a pad of cotton wool soaked in the liquid. Afterwards sprinkle with talcum powder.

NETTLE STINGS

Olive oil

Dab the affected area with a wad of cotton wool soaked in olive oil.

Ox-eye daisies

Rub the afflicted part with fresh ox-eye daisy leaves which have first been rubbed between the hands.

Sorrel

Apply crushed sorrel leaves to the area where the nettles have touched the skin.

Elder leaves

Crush some fresh elder leaves and apply them to the parts that have been stung.

WARTS

Popular medicine has a lot to offer for the treatment of warts. It is difficult to estimate the value of the procedures which may work on some subjects and not on others. Therefore it is sometimes necessary to try several methods in order to find the one that suits the patient.

Garlic method

Apply a small slice of garlic to the wart and fix it in place with sticking plaster. This dressing should preferably be applied before retiring to bed and removed the following morning. Repeat several nights running. The treatment should be stopped after a week even though no visible result seems to have been obtained. After a few days from the cessation of treatment the wart generally drops off. In some parts of France people merely rub the warts with freshly-cut garlic several times a day.

Onion method

Make a hole in the centre of a large onion and fill it with rock salt. Put the onion in a bowl and after 24 hours pour the liquid thus obtained into a bottle. Dab the warts with this preparation in the morning and at night.

Lemon method

Macerate the rind of a lemon in strong vinegar for two days. Cut a piece of rind large enough to cover the wart and place it on the wart at night, holding it in place with sticking plaster. Remove it in the morning and renew the treatment for two further nights.

Another method consists of macerating the rind of two lemons in strong vinegar for a week. With the liquid obtained, the warts should be dabbed twice a day.

Sundry other methods

Fig tree: the following method can only be used in those countries where figs are readily available. Twice daily cut from a fig tree a twig. Apply a small amount of the milky juice exuded to the wart. A green fig may be used in place of the twig.

Salsify or Purple Goatsbeard: rub the warts with a sliced piece of salsify night and morning.
Elder: gather fresh elder leaves. Pound them in a mortar and with the juice obtained dab the warts twice a day.
Peas: rub the warts with fresh green peas cut in half. Give the treatment twice daily.
Thuya or arbor vitae: pour in a flask three coffeespoonfuls of coarsely-chopped thuya leaves and add four tablespoonfuls of alcohol 70°. Macerate for ten days, shaking the flask once a day. Strain and dab the warts with the liquid morning and night.
Marigold: macerate marigold leaves in strong vinegar for two days. Apply a folded leaf to the wart. Hold in place with sticking plaster and leave in place during the night. Repeat the treatment for three consecutive nights.

Another method consists of chopping marigold flowers and applying them in the form of a poultice to the wart. Cover with a compress and secure by sticking plaster and leave in place through the night.
Slugs: although the following method is somewhat off-putting it is said to be most effective, but we have no proof if it works or not. Twice a day find a large slug (they usually hide in damp places, under stones or flower-pots) and rub it on the warts so that they are impregnated with the slug's mucus or slime. If you try this method be sure to hold the slug carefully so as not to injure it and, when used, place it exactly where you found it.
Dandelion: gather some thick dandelion stems and dab the warts with the mulky juice which they exude.

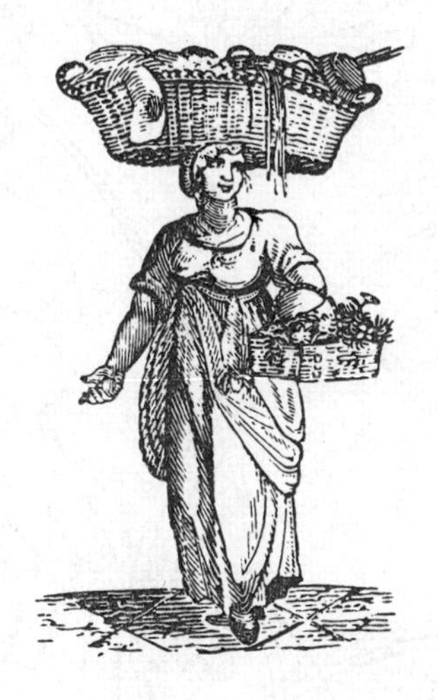

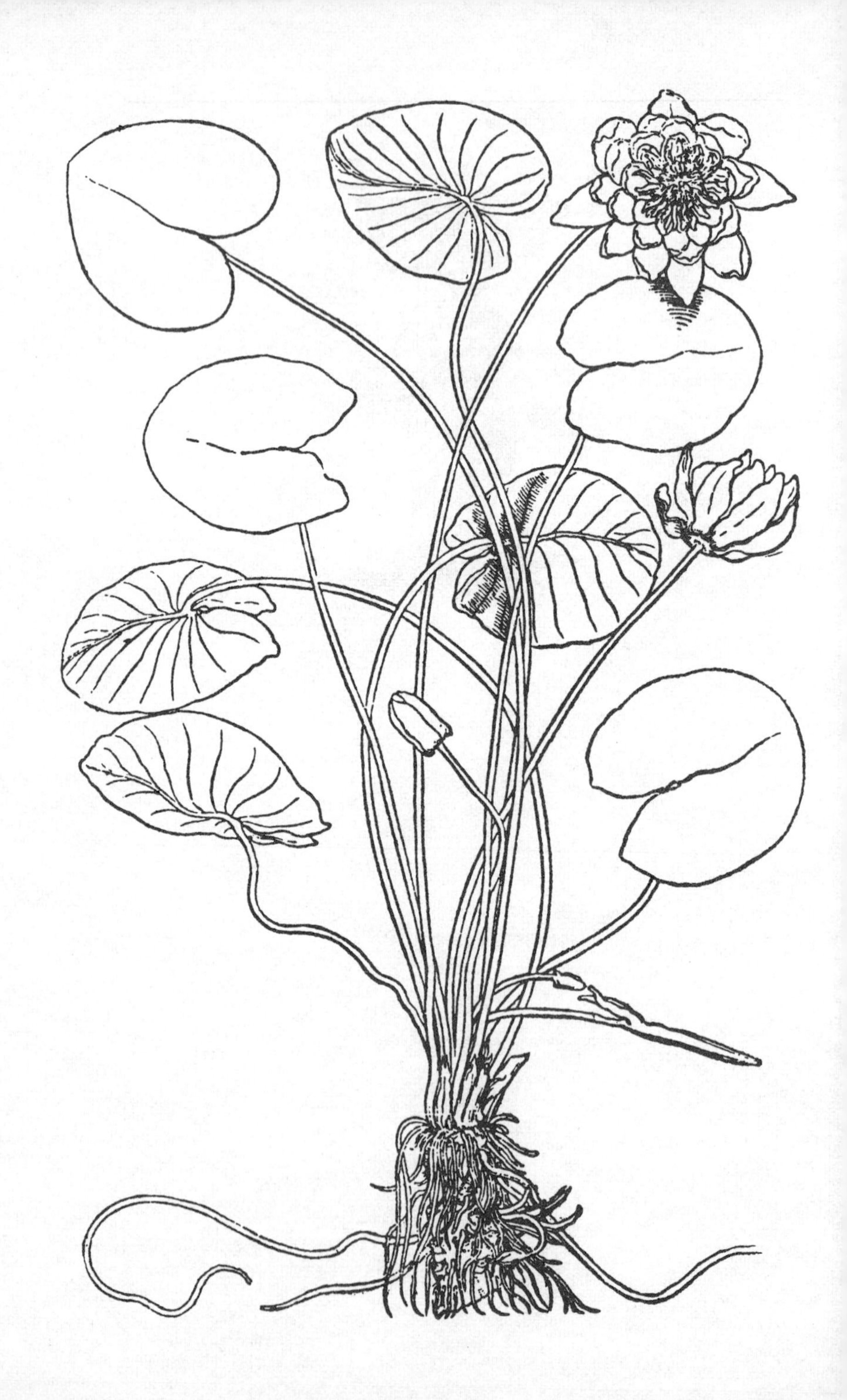

Eyes, Nose, Mouth and Ears

INFLAMMATION OF THE EYES AND EYELIDS

Decoction of cornflower

Use an eyebath and a decoction of cornflower (preparation No. 27) and bathe the eye for three minutes, keeping the eyelid well open. Another method consists of applying compresses soaked in the same decoction and held to the eye for fifteen minutes. The cornflower decoction is always used cold.

Camomile

Put in a cup one tablespoonful of camomile flowers and pour boiling water on them. Cover and leave to infuse for ten minutes. Strain through a fine cloth. Bathe the eyes with the cold infusion twice daily.

Chervil

Apply to the eyelids compresses soaked in cold chervil infusion for a quarter of an hour three times daily (preparation No. 51).

Parsley

Put in the eyes two drops of fresh parsley juice three times daily. One can also apply to the eyelids a compress of crushed parsley leaves. The poultice should be kept in place for half an hour.

Liquorice

Apply twice daily to the eyelids a compress soaked in a tepid infusion of liquorice (preparation No. 135).

IRRITATED EYES

Cabbage juice

Before retiring at night put in the eyes three drops of cabbage juice which should be extracted at the time it is needed.

Maceration of liquorice

Apply to the eyes by means of an eyebath a cold maceration of liquorice (preparation No. 136).

SWOLLEN EYELIDS

Raw potato

Grate some raw peeled potatoes. Wrap the pulp in a gauze compress and apply it to the eyelids. Hold in place for fifteen minutes.

Rose water

Put in a cup one coffeespoonful of cornflowers. Pour on them rose water which has been heated but not boiled. Cover and leave to infuse for a quarter of an hour. Bathe the eyes with the preparation when it has become lukewarm.

Laurel

Boil laurel leaves in wine for ten minutes. Crush the leaves and enclose them in a gauze compress. Apply the compress to the eyes for fifteen minutes.

BLACK EYES

Apple poultice

Apply to the bruised eye a compress of grated apples, wrapped in gauze. Repeat the application once every hour. The small dessert apples called rennets (from the French *reinette*) are considered particularly efficacious.

STYES

Sweet basil

Chop finely some fresh sweet basil. Place it in a compress that has been soaked in rose water; apply the preparation to the affected eye for one hour at least.

Infusion of elder

Place in a receptable a glassful of elder flowers (either fresh or dried flowers may be used). Pour on them a litre of boiling water. Cover and leave to infuse for ten minutes. Strain through a cloth and wash the stye with the cold preparation at least five times daily.

Sundry methods

Pork fat: take a slice of raw pork rind and apply the inner surface to the eye. Cover with a gauze compress and retain for an hour.
Garlic: rub lightly with the raw part of a cut clove of garlic.
Veal: apply to the eye a small piece of raw veal held by a compress. Keep it there for an hour.

SQUINTS

We offer the following treatment for squints without, however, having any direct knowledge or proof of its effectiveness. When it is noticed that a child has a tendency to squint, cover the unaffected eye with a black bandage so that for a month the child uses only the eye that squints. Then reverse the procedure so that it is the normal eye only that is used. Remove the bandage after three weeks; the squint, provided it was not too acute, should have been corrected.

DEFECTIVE EYESIGHT

According to popular belief some eyesight disorders can be alleviated and shortsightedness diminished by drinking a cup of wild carrot decoction (preparation No. 47).

NOSE BLEEDING

Cold footbath

Take a footbath in water at a temperature of about 10°C. Even though the bleeding may have stopped keep your feet in the water until either the legs ache or there is a sensation of warmth.

Cold compress

Place on the nape of the neck very cold compresses which are renewed every five minutes.

Constriction method

Bind fairly tightly with thin string two fingers of the right hand. Likewise bind the left forearm. Apparently this method is often very efficacious but should not be prolonged beyond five minutes.

Sundry treatments

Vinegar: put in the ears three drops of vinegar (if the bleeding occurs in one nostril only, restrict the drops to the ear on the same side).
Lemon: place in each nostril a small piece of cotton wool soaked in lemon juice.
Shepherd's purse wine: inhale through each nostril a few drops of shepherd's purse wine (preparation No. 36a).
Nettles: extract the juice of fresh stinging nettle leaves and stalks. Soak two small pieces of cotton wool in the juice and place in the nostrils.

SINUSITIS

Caster sugar
Sniff through both nostrils a small quantity of very fine sugar, such as caster sugar, three or four times a day.

Camomile inhalation
Prepare an infusion of camomile (preparation No. 45) and inhale it twice a day, draping a thick towel over the head and the infusion jar in order to concentrate the vapour.

APHTHAS (Small mouth ulcers)

Eating is sometimes made painful and difficult by small ulcers on the inside surface of the lips. Popular medicine considers bilberries as the specific treatment for this condition.

Bilberry method
If bilberries are readily available the best method is to pick some and chew them, keeping them in the mouth for as long as possible. Bilberry jam may also be used as a substitute. The efficacy of this treatment may be improved by preparing a decoction of bilberry in the following way: place in a saucepan ten tablespoonfuls of fresh or dried bilberries to a litre of cold water; bring slowly to the boil and maintain at boiling point until the liquid has been reduced to half the original amount; strain, pressing the bilberries well. Use the decoction lukewarm as a mouthwash several times a day.

Other methods
Honey: dissolve a generous tablespoonful of honey in the juice of a lemon. Take a coffeespoonful of the preparation, holding it in the mouth on the sore spots for as long as possible.
Violets: using a lukewarm decoction of violets as a mouthwash (preparation No. 167), proceed as above.
Sage: a warm sage decoction (preparation No. 144) is used as a mouthwash every two hours.
Cornflower: use a decoction, in the same way as above, of corn-

flower, following preparation No. 27, four times a day.
Crane's bill: use a decoction of crane's bill (preparation No. 23) as a mouthwash half an hour before meals. The liquid, which should be used warm, should be kept in the mouth as long as possible. Drink a cup of decoction of white deadnettles and mallow (preparation No. 102) after each mouthwash.

ULCERATIONS OF THE MOUTH

According to popular tradition minor ulcerations of the mouth can be cured either by gargling with wine or by dabbing the affected areas with a cotton bud soaked in Samaritan balm (preparation No. 117).

FEVER SPOTS

Dabbing the fever spots with warm vinegar is considered the best method of getting rid of them, provided it is done properly.

TOOTHACHE

The following methods, like most of those employed in popular medicine, can work with some people but not with others. Even though the pain is reduced no time should be lost in consulting a dentist.

Pepper

Put in a very small receptable two coffeespoonfuls of granulated sugar, one coffeespoonful of ground pepper and a little *eau de vie.* Heat slowly until a caramel is obtained and then pour the caramel on a piece of thick paper. Allow it to cool and then break off a piece about the size of a grain of wheat and apply it to the gum near the affected tooth.

Onion

When a decayed tooth gives pain place in the cavity a small piece of cotton wool soaked in onion juice.

Salt

A salt mouthwash can sometimes relieve toothache. Put a coffee-cupful of rock salt into a large glass of water. Stir until it dissolves and use as a mouthwash.

Poppy

Put in a large cup one tablespoonful of dried poppy flowers and fill with boiling water. Cover and leave to infuse for ten minutes. Strain and use as a mouthwash.

Turnip

Cook a turnip in the oven. Crush it and place it in two small pieces of gauze to be applied as a poultice behind the ears.

Elder

Boil two tablespoonfuls of elder leaves to half a litre of water for ten minutes then strain. Inhale the vapour while keeping the mouth open.

Eau de vie

Use *eau de vie* as a mouthwash several times a day.

Cabbage

Pass a hot iron over several cabbage leaves. Apply two or three layers of them to the cheek.

Nettles

Pound fresh stinging nettles, sprinkling them with table salt. Apply a little of this praparation to the gum close to the affected tooth.

TO REDUCE THE SWELLING OF A GUMBOIL

Rose water butter

Melt 50 g of butter in a saucepan; remove pan from the heat and add a tablespoonful of rose water to the melted butter. When cool apply a little of the preparation to the swollen cheek and repeat the application as soon as the last layer has hardened.

INFLAMMATION OF THE GUMS

Decoction of wood avens (common avens or herb bennet)
Use avens decoction (preparation No. 24) as a mouthwash several times a day.

Liquorice
Put in a saucepan 200 g of liquorice root to a litre of cold water. Bring slowly to the boil and keep it boiling for twenty minutes and then leave to infuse for a quarter of an hour before straining. Twice a day use the preparation lukewarm as a mouthwash.

Oak bark
Use a decoction of oak bark (preparation No. 58) as a mouthwash three times a day.

Lemon juice
Massage the gums, avoiding the teeth, with a piece of cotton wool soaked in lemon juice morning and night.

Quince wine
Use as a mouthwash three times a day lukewarm quince wine (preparation No. 64).

Watercress
Chew thoroughly some watercress, swilling it around the gums.

Salted wine
Massage the gums several times a day with a piece of cotton wool soaked in salted wine – half a coffeespoonful of salt to a glass of red wine.

Sage
Use an infusion of sage (preparation No. 145) as a mouthwash several times a day.

Figwort
Chew thoroughly some fresh figwort.

Veronica
Use a lukewarm decoction of veronica (preparation No. 161) twice a day as a mouthwash.

Violets
Use as set out above a lukewarm decoction of violets (preparation No. 167).

THRUSH

Application of lemon juice
Soak in lemon juice a cotton wool bud and dab the patches of thrush three times a day. Use a fresh cotton wool bud for each affected area.

Mallow infusion
Put in a receptacle one and a half tablespoonfuls of mallow leaves. Pour on half a litre of boiling water. Stir well, cover and leave to infuse for ten minutes. Strain. Drink a cup of this infusion after lunch and another one after dinner.

Mouthwashes
Cornflower: use a warm decoction of cornflowers (preparation No. 27) as a mouthwash six times a day.
*Sage:*proceed as above, using a hot sage decoction instead of cornflower (preparation No. 144).

HALITOSIS

Bad breath my be caused by eating strong-smelling food or may have a pathological origin.

The undermentioned procedures are only intended to deal with halitosis itself. Even if satisfactory results are obtained by following one of the treatments it is recommended that the patient seek a doctor's or a dentist's advice to discover the cause.

Coffee bean method

The following method is considered particularly efficacious when bad breath has been caused by eating raw onions. Take three coffee beans, crunch and chew them thoroughly for fifteen minutes, taking care to swill the pieces thoroughly into all the corners of the mouth. Spit out and drink a glass of water.

Parsley method

The following method is particularly efficacious for bad breath caused by eating garlic. Chew a sprig of parsley slowly for a quarter of an hour. Then spit it out and eat an apple.

Sundry methods

Peroxide of hydrogen: mix three tablespoonfuls of peroxide of hydrogen with ten tablespoonfuls of distilled water. Pour two tablespoonfuls of this preparation into half a glass of warm water. Rinse the mouth thoroughly.

Wood avens: as a mouthwash use a decoction of wood avens (preparation No. 24) hot and unsweetened.

Cornflower: use as a mouthwash a lukewarm and unsweetened decoction of cornflowers (preparation No. 27).

Camomile: after having made a strong infusion of camomile (preparation No. 45) mix it with an equal quantity of glycerine. Use it lukewarm as a mouthwash and then rinse profusely with cold water.

Black radish (Raphanus niger): chew leaves of black radish for fifteen minutes. Spit out and rinse the mouth in cold water.

HARDNESS OF HEARING

According to popular beliefs hearing can be improved by inserting into the ears a small wad of cotton wool soaked in garlic juice. Apply each night. The same therapeutic property is attributed to cabbage and lemon juice which should be mixed in equal quantities and a few drops put into the ears.

BUZZING IN THE EAR

Oil of apricot stones

Crack some apricot stones and remove the almonds which are then crushed in a mortar. With the oil thus obtained the ears are treated by putting in a few drops every morning.

Onion juice

Insert in the ear a small piece of cotton wool soaked in onion juice.

Infusion of balm

Drink four cups of infusion of balm (preparation No. 104) after each of the three main meals of the day and one at bedtime.

Vinegar

Put in a small receptacle some boiling vinegar. Place an inverted funnel over it and place the ear to the spout so that the vapour penetrates the ear.

INSECT IN THE EAR

Warm oil method

Get the patient to lie down on the side opposite to that of the affected ear. After having warmed some olive oil (make sure that it is not too hot and test the temperature by putting a drop of oil on the back of the hand) place a few drops in the infected ear. More often than not the insect will come out immediately.

EARACHE

It is not clear in popular medicine what is meant by earache. Therefore the undermentioned treatments should be considered with caution and ignored altogether in a case that seems to be serious.

Olive oil

Put in the ear a small piece of cotton wool soaked in lukewarm olive oil.

Onion

Cook a small onion in the oven. When soft it should be mashed with a little butter, enclosed in gauze and placed in the ear.

Garlic

Grate a piece of garlic and enclose it in a piece of gauze which is then introduced into the painful ear.

Parsley

Chop finely some parsley and mash together with a little olive oil so as to obtain a pellet that can be inserted in the ear. *(Translator's note:* The French original says nothing about using a piece of gauze but it is safer to do so rather than introduce chopped vegetable matter without a wrapping. In any case, do not make the pellet so small that it goes so far into the ear that it is difficult to extract.)

Lily oil

Place in the affected ear a small cotton wool pad permeated with lily oil (preparation No. 97).

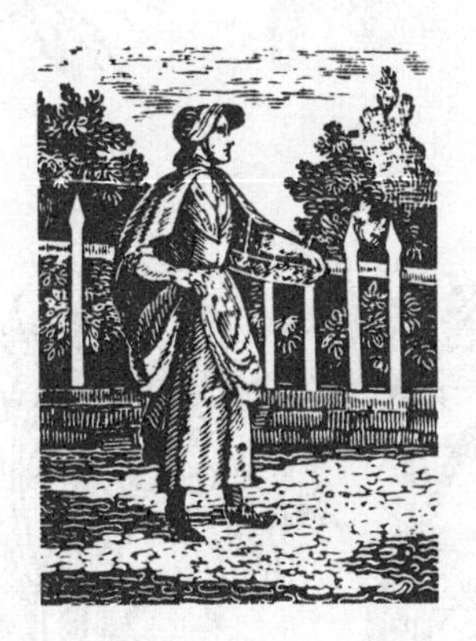

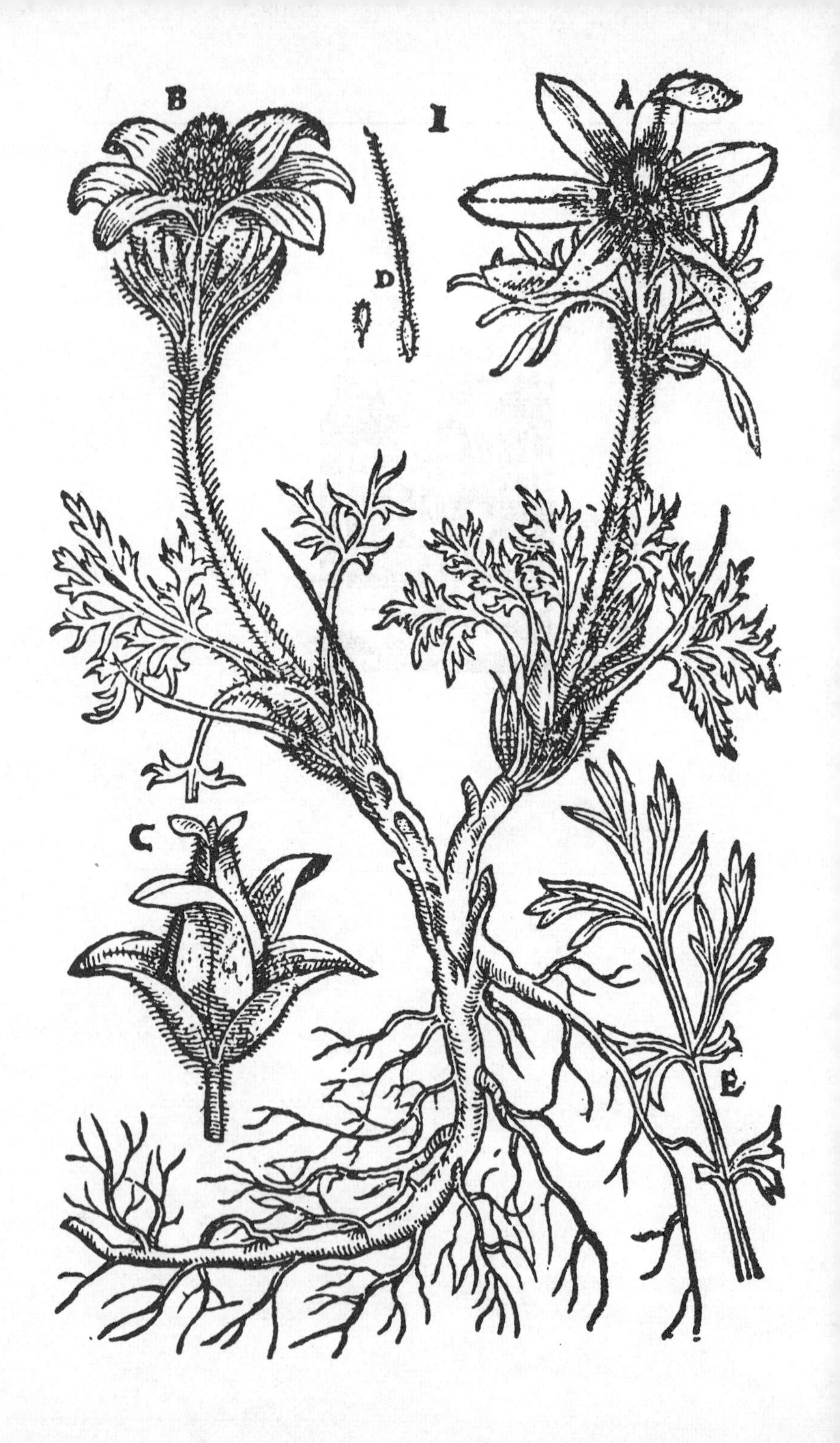
B
I
A
D
C
E

Hands and Feet

CORNS · CHILBLAINS · WALKER'S FATIGUE
BRITTLE AND FRAGILE FINGERNAILS · WHITLOWS
EXCESSIVE FOOT PERSPIRATION

CORNS

There is no distinction made in popular medicine between different types of foot callosities and therefore the methods used to treat corns can also be applied to any other kind of thickened skin.

Garlic method

Take a footbath for a quarter of an hour and then apply to the healthy skin around the corn pieces of sticking plaster. Crush well a piece of garlic and spread the pulp on the corn. Cover with several layers of gauze held in place by sticking plaster.

Keep the dressing in place throughout the night and repeat every evening until relief is obtained.

In certain regions of France garlic which has been cooked in the oven is used instead.

Sundry methods

Ivy: first macerate some ivy leaves in white vinegar for four days. Cut a few pieces of ivy leaves to the size of the corn. Cover the corn with several layers of ivy and hold them in place with a gauze compress and sticking plaster. Keep the dressing in place for three days and then take a very hot footbath. It should now be easy to remove the corn but if it is not repeat the treatment for three more days. Sometimes the removal of a corn is obtained by merely rubbing it with ivy leaves prepared as set out above.

Leek: first macerate a green leaf of a leek in a good white wine vinegar for twenty-four hours. Take care to choose a good thick leaf.

At night, after taking a footbath for fifteen minutes, apply to the corn a piece of leek which does not overlap the healthy sur-

rounding skin. Cover with a gauze compress held by sticking plaster. Take another footbath the following morning and renew the treatment every night until the corn is detached.
Meadow saffron: using a pestle and mortar, crush some fresh meadow saffron leaves.

At night, after taking a footbath, cover the healthy skin surrounding the corn with sticking plaster. Place on the corn a small quantity of the crushed leaves and cover with a gauze compress held firmly in place. Keep the dressing there for twenty-four hours and repeat the treatment for five days. If after this time there seems to be no visible change, do not worry, as the corn will drop off of its own accord a few days later.

CHILBLAINS

Chilblains are a very painful inflammation affecting mostly the fingers and toes. They are brought on by the cold and people with circulatory disorders or those who are undernourished are particularly prone to them. This is why popular medicine advises those suffering from chilblains to eat a lot of uncooked vegetables and drink plenty of fresh fruit juice.

According to tradition a preventive measure which we have not had occasion to check at first hand is to rub the hands with crushed strawberries, when they are in season, for a quarter of an hour each day.

Chervil method

Chop coarsely 500 g of fresh chervil (if fresh chervil is not available use dried chervil). Put it in a basin with a litre of vinegar and 400 g of rock salt. Leave to macerate for two hours, stirring from time to time. Soak the hands in this preparation three times a day for a quarter of an hour. The preparation can be used for a few consecutive days provided a little vinegar is added each day to maintain the level of the liquid.

Celeriac method

Cut into small pieces a kilo of celeriac and put it into a receptacle with four litres of cold water. Bring slowly to the boil, boil for one hour. Strain the liquid. Soak the hands or feet, as the need may be, twice a day in this decoction for a quarter of an hour. The water should be as hot as is bearable. Dry well with a towel and put on immediately woollen gloves or socks which should be worn constantly, day and night.

Turnip method

Cook in the oven a large unpeeled turnip. As soon as it is soft allow it to cool and then cut in half. Rub the chilblain vigorously with the cut surface. This treatment is best followed before retiring at night.

Sundry methods

Alum: melt 100 g of mutton fat. Mix thoroughly the liquid fat with a coffeespoonful of powdered alum and pour into a jar. Leave to cool. Dab the chilblains twice a day with this ointment.
Spirit of salt: dab the chilblains with a piece of cotton wool soaked with spirit of salt; apply the treatment three or four times a day. This procedure is only possible when there are no cracks or chapping present.
Lemon: rub the chilblains with a piece of cotton soaked with lemon juice, applying several times a day.
Garlic: rub the chilblains several times a day with the cut surface of a clove of garlic.
Cabbage: crush with a rolling pin the leaves of a cabbage; apply pieces of leaves to the chilblains and hold in place with narrow strips of crêpe. Repeat with new leaves every three hours.
Cornflour: mix well in a basin 500 g of cornflour with an equal amount of sawdust. Plunge the hands into the mixture, rubbing well the affected areas two or three times a day for fifteen-minute periods.
Chicken gall bladder: ask a poulterer or butcher for a dozen gall bladders removed from chicken livers. Put 100 g of lard into a receptacle, hold the gall bladders over it and pierce them. Mix

the gall well with the lard and rub the ointment on the chilblains morning and night.
Mistletoe: put in a receptacle 200 g of chopped mistletoe leaves to two litres of cold water. Bring slowly to the boil, cook for one hour and strain.

Bathe hands or feet for ten minutes twice or thrice daily each day in the concoction which should be heated at the time of use to the maximum temperature that can be borne. Afterwards, quickly rinse with cold water and massage with a little olive oil.
Juniper: place some juniper berries into a hot frying-pan and expose the chilblains to the vapour arising from them.
Kidney beans: cook, for three-quarters of the usual time allowed when the beans are to be eaten, 500 g of kidney beans in three litres of water. Soak the hands for a quarter of an hour several times a day in the liquid which must be reheated each time it is used.
Soot: collect a glassful of soot from the chimney and stir it into a litre of vinegar. Rub the hands well with the preparation three times a day.
Candle wax: to calm the discomfort of chilblains hold a lighted candle above them and allow the melted was to fall on them. Leave the patches of wax until they fall of their own accord.
Vine leaves: bathe hands or feet in a warm decoction of vine leaves (preparation No. 166).
Marigold: bathe hands or feet in a lukewarm infusion of marigold (preparation No. 150) three times a day for a quarter of an hour.
Oak bark: bathe hands or feet for a quarter of an hour four times a day in a lukewarm decoction of oak bark (preparation No. 58).

WALKER'S FATIGUE

Preventive measures

According to popular tradition the tiring effects of a long walk can be lessened by putting fresh mugwort leaves in the shoes before setting out. If fresh leaves are not available use dried mugwort leaves which have been dipped in water and dried for a few minutes between two sheets of blotting paper.

Cold footbath

The tiring effects of a long walk may be lessened by bathing the feet in cold water. Soak the feet in the water which should not be warmer than 10°C. and keep the feet in the water until there is a sensation of warmth or the feet ache. The result may be one or the other according to the individual. Dry well and put on woollen socks.

BRITTLE AND FRAGILE NAILS

Olive oil method

Mix olive oil – half a coffeecupful – with the juice of half a lemon. Heat well but not to boiling point.

Dab the nails with a cotton wool pad soaked in the mixture. After about a minute rub the nails against one another. Repeat the treatment three of four times each day until there is an improvement and then continue the treatment once a week.

Sundry methods

Lemon: apply to the nails the juice of a lemon morning and night for one week.

Pork: rub the nails with pork rind or crackling morning and night.

Watercress: crush well some watercress seeds and mix them with a little honey until a thick paste is obtained. Apply a little of this paste to the nails each night. Apply dressings and leave them in place until next morning.

WHITLOWS

A whitlow is an inflammation close to a nail. It is often the result of the fingertip being pricked by a needle or thorn. The inflammation gives acute pain which can last for several weeks unless it is treated. The methods suggested by popular medicine help considerably in lessening the intensity and duration of the pain.

Egg method

This treatment is applied before retiring at night. Make a hole in the shell of a fresh egg and place the infected finger in it, making sure that the whitlow is in the yolk. Fix with sticking plaster to ensure that the finger remains inside the egg and to prevent the raw egg from running out. Wrap the hand in soft cloths and towels so that the eggshell is not broken during the night. If this method if followed correctly the whitlow should have been healed by the following morning.

Other treatments

Hawthorn: peel the bark from some hawthorn branches, taking care to choose those areas that are particularly resinous. Heat the pieces of bark in a *bain marie* (double saucepan) after crushing them as much as possible while they are cooking. Apply the paste obtained direct to the whitlow and cover with a piece of gauze held in place by a small bandage.
Onion: cook an onion in the oven. When it is soft mash it with a fork to an even paste which is then applied to the whitlow. Cover with a piece of gauze held by a bandage. Repeat the treatment night and morning.
Greater celandine: apply several fresh leaves of greater celandine to the whitlow. Cover with gauze and fix in place.
Bramble: crush finely, using a pestle and mortar, fresh bramble leaves. Wrap the crushed leaves in a small piece of gauze and apply the compress to the whitlow. Hold the dressing in place with a bandage. Repeat two or three times a day.

EXCESSIVE FOOT PERSPIRATION

Pine needle bath

Toss into two litres of water a kilo of pine or fir tree needles. Leave it to boil for ten minutes and strain, pressing the mixture well. Take a footbath in this decoction for fifteen minutes in the morning.

Sundry methods

Tincture of horsetail: each morning dab the feet (paying particular attention to the toes and soles) with tincture of horsetail (preparation No. 132).

Alder tree leaves: according to popular tradition if fresh alder leaves are placed inside the shoes and kept there while the shoes are worn they will discourage excessive sweating of the feet.

Hemp leaves: crush between the hands fresh hemp leaves and rub into the feet the liquid exuded by the leaves.

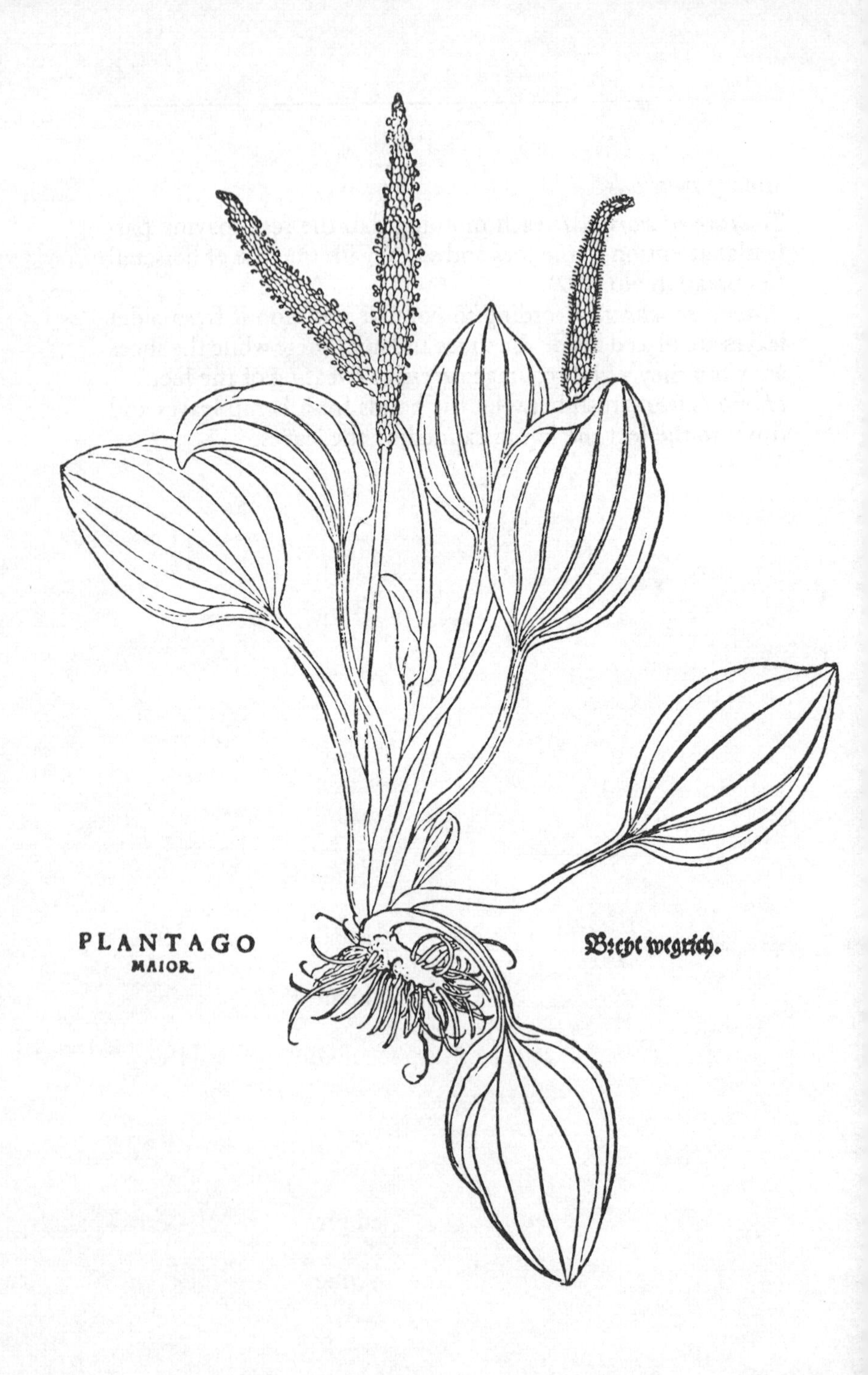
PLANTAGO
MAIOR
Breyt wegrich.

Pains affecting Muscles, Joints and Nerve Points

ARTHRITIS · STIFFNESS · MUSCULAR CRAMP
INTERCOSTAL PAINS · SPRAINS AND TWISTS OF THE ANKLE
GOUT · LUMBAGO · NEURALGIA · NEURITIS · STITCH
RHEUMATISM · SCIATICA · STIFF NECK

ARTHRITIS

Laurel leaf lotion

Put in a saucepan three handfuls of laurel leaves and the same quantity of nettle leaves and marshmallow. Add three litres of cold water, bring to the boil slowly and simmer for three hours. Strain and rub the affected part with the lotion three times a day.

Other methods

Artichoke: drink three cupfuls of artichoke infusion daily: one before breakfast, one an hour before lunch and another one before the evening meal (preparation No. 15). Follow the treatment every day for a fortnight.
Clematis: massage the painful spots three times a day with clematis alcohol (preparation No. 62).
Blackcurrant: drink four cups daily of decoction of blackcurrant leaves (preparation No. 49), namely, one before breakfast, one before lunch, one between lunch and dinner and a fourth before retiring to bed.
Meadowsweet: before each of the three main meals drink a cup of meadowsweet infusion (preparation No. 137).

STIFFNESS

If stiffness is the result of unaccustomed physical effort, drink a claret glass of onion wine (preparation No. 116). If the stiffness is a regular affliction, take a cure of onion wine, namely, one claret glass before breakfast each day.

MUSCULAR CRAMP

Popular medicine treats cramp with water, either icy cold or very hot.

According to the spot where the cramp occurs treat with icy cold water, either under a shower or by a compress.

If the hot compress method is preferred add some vinegar to the water in the proportion of one coffeecup to half a litre of boiling water. These compresses should be applied as hot as possible, taking care not to scald the skin.

Writer's cramp is treated in the following way: fill a basin with water at a temperature of 40–50 °C. Place the folded arms in the water and keep them there for ten minutes. Dry the arms by rubbing them briskly with a towel.

Sundry treatments

Melilot: as soon as cramp is felt drink a cup of melilot infusion (preparation No. 103).

If frequently affected by cramp, drink during one week of every month four cupfuls of the infusion: one cup first thing in the morning, one cup in the course of the morning, another in the afternoon and a fourth at night before retiring.

Nettles: rub with fresh stinging nettles the affected muscles.

Tansy: as soon as cramp is felt drink a cup of tansy infusion (preparation No. 153).

Thyme: the infusion described below has the reputation of being particularly efficacious.

Place in a receptacle half a coffeespoonful of thyme, six heads of camomile, a small coffeespoonful of fennel seeds, a small coffeespoonful of goosefoot, a generous coffeespoonful of lime flowers and a similar amount of mint leaves. Pour on a litre of boiling water. Stir well, leave covered for ten minutes to infuse. Strain.

Drink a cupful of the infusion as soon as possible after the onset of the cramp, then drink a second cup half an hour later and after a further lapse of one hour drink a third.

INTERCOSTAL PAINS

To ease the pain, rub the places affected with clematis alcohol (preparation No. 62).

SPRAINS AND STRAINS

Mugwort poultice

Pound thoroughly in a mortar some fresh mugwort leaves. Wrap in gauze and apply to the sprain, holding the dressing in place with a bandage. Renew the poultice every four hours.

Camomile oil

Apply to the swelling compresses permeated with camomile oil (preparation No. 43) and keep in place in the appropriate manner. Repeat every three hours.

Cabbage leaves

Apply to the affected limb four layers of cabbage leaves (see preparation No. 55). Cover with a generous wad of cotton wool and keep in place with a dressing which should not be too tight. Retain the poultice throughout the day and replace with a fresh one at night.

Thistle compress

Put in a receptacle six tablespoonfuls of dried thistle leaves to a litre of cold water. Bring slowly to the boil, simmer for a quarter of an hour and strain. Apply to the swelling compresses that have been soaked in the lukewarm decoction and repeat the treatment every three hours.

Roots of comfrey

Grate some comfrey roots and then steep them in olive oil as though you were making a green salad. Then wrap up the preparation in gauze. Apply to the affected limb and fix with a bandage or similar dressing. Retain the poultice all day and repeat the treatment in the evening.

Wine of bittersweet

Put in a saucepan ten tablespoonfuls of bittersweet leaves together with a litre of red wine. Bring slowly to the boil, boil for ten minutes and strain. Apply to the injury lukewarm compresses soaked in the preparation and repeat the treatment every two hours.

Infusion of tansy

Apply to the affected limb compresses soaked with tansy infusion (preparation No. 153) and hold in place with an appropriate dressing. Repeat every four hours.

Moss poultice

Gather some moss from the bole of a tree or close to a rock. Soak the moss in water and, without wringing out the water, apply it to the swelling at once; cover with a strip of gauze held in position by a dressing. Repeat once in the morning and once at night.

GOUT

In the past gout was a common affliction and scarce were the families whose members had not sought treatment for it at one time or another. Therefore the methods employed for the treatment of gout by popular medicine have been improved from generation to generation. As a result, the methods are often most satisfactory. According to popular tradition, gouty people should eat a lot of fruit, vegetables and milky foods; alcohol and spices are not recommended.

Ointment of garlic and houseleek

Pound finely in a mortar equal quantities of garlic cloves and fresh houseleek leaves. Spread the mash on the painful area, cover with gauze and hold in place with a dressing. Keep the poultice on throughout the night.

Rosemary lotion

Put in a container (popular tradition advises the use of an earthenware receptacle such as a jug) ten tablespoonfuls of blackcurrant leaves, the same quantity of sage leaves and likewise ten tablespoonfuls of rosemary; add a litre of white wine, cover and leave to macerate in a warm place for twenty-four hours, stirring from time to time the mixture with a wooden spoon. After that filter and pour into a bottle.

When the lotion is used heat only the quantity needed for one treatment and massage the painful areas with the preparation, which should be applied very warm, several times a day.

Other methods

Cornflower: take a small glass of cornflower wine (preparation No. 28) before breakfast, one before lunch and one at night before retiring.

Birch: chop some fresh birch leaves and make a poultice with them which is then applied to the painful spots. At the same time, drink an infusion of birch leaves (preparation No. 32) four times a day: a cupful half an hour before the midday meal, another two hours after lunch, a third half an hour before the evening meal and the last two hours after having eaten.

Borage: when in pain drink four cups of borage decoction (preparation No. 35) leaving intervals of twenty minutes between each draught.

Camomile: cook for ten minutes a handful of camomile flowers; wrap the flowers in gauze of suitable dimensions and apply the poultice to the tender area. One can also rub oil of camomile (preparation No. 43) on the site of the pain.

Turnip; cook in the oven a turnip. Mash it with a fork and apply the purée to the painful area. Cover with gauze held in place with a dressing. Keep the poultice on until it is completely cold.

Medlar: place in a litre bottle 100 g of crushed medlar stones; fill with white wine, cork and leave to macerate for twenty-four hours, shaking the bottle from time to time. Filter and pour into the storage bottle. Drink an aperitif glass of this wine before breakfast. One bottle should last for a month.

Strawberries: according to popular tradition gouty people should take a cure of strawberries throughout the season when they are available. One pound should be eaten during the day, in the following amounts: half a pound first thing in the morning and another half a pound at some time between the midday and evening meals.
Horseradish: from the moment a gout attack starts drink a cupful before breakfast of horseradish decoction (preparation No. 133) for ten consecutive days.
Thyme: drink during the gout attack an infusion of thyme in a large cup (preparation No. 156).

LUMBAGO

Medlar wine

Place in a litre bottle 100 g of medlar stones and top up with white wine. Leave to macerate for twenty-four hours, shaking the bottle five or six times. Filter while transferring from one bottle to another.

Drink first thing in the morning, when suffering from lumbago, an aperitif glass of this wine.

Bryony massage

Obtain some fresh white bryony roots, preferably shortly before they are to be used. Cut crosswise a piece of root and massage with the cut surface the painful area. If a repetition of the treatment is needed ensure that another freshly-cut section of root is used. Do not dry the skin after the massage but cover the area with a piece of warm flannel.

Other methods

Hemp: wind a length of hemp string around the waist and loins so as to form a kind of corset.
Greater celandine: drink three cupfuls of greater celandine infusion (preparation No. 54a): one cup before breakfast, one before lunch and one before going to bed.

Onions: during the course of the lumbago attack drink, first thing in the morning, a glass of onion wine (preparation No. 116).
Thyme: pour into a container a strong infusion of thyme (preparation No. 156) and expose the painful areas to the vapour arising from it.

NEURALGIA

Nettles

A most efficient method of treating neuralgia, according to popular medicine, is to rub the painful spots with stinging nettles immediately they have been gathered.

Mistletoe wine

Put in a receptacle two tablespoonfuls of mistletoe leaves, twelve flower heads of camomile, and four tablespoonfuls of maidenhair fern. Add a litre of white wine, cover and allow to macerate for five days, stirring twice a day. Strain and decant. Drink a glass of this wine after each of the principal meals.

Mullein alcohol

Place in a litre bottle three tablespoonfuls of mullein flowers; fill up the bottle with alcohol 90° and seal. Leave to macerate for ten days, shaking the bottle twice a day. At the end of that time strain and transfer to another bottle. Rub the painful areas twice a day with the preparation.

Other methods

Camomile: when in pain, drink a large cupful of camomile infusion (preparation No. 44).
Cabbage: cook some cabbage leaves slowly in milk, stirring constantly until the leaves have been reduced to a pulp. Wrap the preparation in gauze of an appropriate size and apply to the sore area.

Another method consists of pressing some cabbage leaves with a lukewarm iron (after having removed the larger ribs) and then placing them on the painful spots.

Ash: before each of the main meals drink a cup of ash leaf infusion (preparation No. 83).
Lettuce: when in pain drink a cup of lettuce leaf decoction (preparation No. 93).
Leeks: put in a saucepan the white part of three leeks that have been chopped into pieces, three garlic cloves, sprinkle generously with salt and add just enough water to cover them. Cook slowly until the liquid has completely evaporated; wrap the preparation in gauze of suitable size and apply to the painful area.
Elder: when in pain, drink a cup of infusion of elder flowers (preparation No. 152).
Thyme: when in pain drink – but not too soon after meals – a cup of thyme infusion (preparation No. 156).
Verbena: prepare a decoction of verbena (preparation No. 164). When it has cooled soak compresses with it and apply them to the painful areas. This method is particularly recommended for facial neuralgia.

NEURITIS

As a palliative for neuritis, popular medicine recommends a friction with clematis alcohol (preparation No. 62).

STITCH

The specific popular remedy for stitch is the juice that has been squeezed out of chervil to fill half a glass which is then topped up with the same amount of white wine. Two hours should elapse between drinking the wine and taking any food.

Other methods

Leeks: place in a frying-pan two chopped leeks; sprinkle generously with salt and just cover with vinegar. Cook very slowly, stirring until all the vinegar has evaporated. Wrap the leeks in

gauze and apply to the painful place in the side and cover with a flannel cloth.
Valerian: drink before each of the main meals a cupful of valerian infusion (preparation No. 160).
Oats: put in a saucepan two handfuls of oats to half a glass of vinegar. Stirring well, heat the preparation and apply it wrapped in gauze and covered with flannel. *(Translator's note:* oats in the form in which they are given to horses are almost certainly intended here but coarse oatmeal or even packet porridge oats (readily available in the U.K. but rare in France) will do as substitutes.
Verbena: apply a verbena poultice (preparation No. 163) and also drink three times a day before meals a cupful of verbena decoction (preparation No. 164).

RHEUMATISM

Thyme poultice

Heat, without adding anything, in a saucepan or frying-pan sprigs of thyme. Wrap the thyme in a piece of gauze of suitable size and apply to the painful areas. Cover with a piece of flannel and maintain the poultice for as long as it remains hot.

Bag of birch leaves method

To ease rheumatic pains in an arm or leg fill with fresh birch leaves a bag or sack into which the limb in need of treatment is inserted and left for at least two hours.

Popular medicine also recommends as a method of keeping at bay rheumatism the use of a mattress filled with birch leaves, elder leaves or fern leaves. Whichever leaves are chosen should be lightly dried in the oven before use.

Fennel wine

Put in a container a coffeespoonful of fennel leaves, a coffeespoonful of verbena leaves, a coffeespoonful of lime leaves, half a grated nutmeg and a litre of red wine. Cover and allow to macerate throughout the night before straining. Drink an aperitif glass of the preparation first thing in the morning, one glass before lunch and another before retiring at night.

Lemon cure

This method has long had a reputation of being very effective but we have no personal knowledge of its action.

Drink on the first day of the cure the juice of two lemons. On the second day, drink the juice of four lemons (taken in two doses). On the third day the juice of six lemons (taken in three doses) – and so on until the juice of twenty lemons is being taken in ten doses on the tenth day of the cure. On the eleventh day reduce the dose by two lemons, on the twelfth by two more and carry on until the nineteenth and last day is reached.

Cabbage poultice

Melt some lard in a *bain marie* and when it is thoroughly hot plunge into it some cabbage leaves. Remove them after a few seconds, let them drain a little and then wrap them in a piece of gauze cut to the appropriate size. Apply to the painful area.

Sage bath

Enclose in a muslin sachet 200 g of sage, 200 g of thyme and 200 g of mint leaves. Place them in a receptacle containing four litres of boiling water and boil for a quarter of an hour. Add the preparation to the water of a hot bath. Lie in the bath for twenty minutes. On getting out of the bath empty the sachet of its contents and with them give yourself a brisk massage. Without drying yourself put on a dressing gown and lie down in a warm place for half an hour.

Leek broth

Cook in a litre of unsalted water two large leeks that have been cut into slices, a large onion cut into segments and three pieces of garlic. Strain. Drink the total liquid obtained during the course of the day, taking it in a number of draughts. Follow this treatment for one week.

Sundry other methods

Garlic: place in a bottle ten grated cloves of garlic; add one quarter of a litre of 90° alcohol and leave to macerate for one month, shaking the bottle every day. Strain. Take before the midday and evening meals half a coffeespoonful of the preparation in a little water.

Mugwort: put into a receptacle 200 g of mugwort leaves to four litres of cold water. Bring to the boil, boil for a quarter of an hour, strain and add the decoction to the water of a hot bath.

Artichoke: take before each of the three main meals a tablespoonful of artichoke maceration (preparation No. 16).

Cornflower: drink before each of the three main meals an aperitif glass of cornflower wine (preparation No. 28).

Birch: drink an infusion of birch leaves (preparation No. 32): four cupfuls daily, namely: one cup to be taken two hours after breakfast, one two hours after the midday meal, one cup half an hour before the evening meal and the last one before retiring to bed.

Borage: during rheumatic attacks drink four cups of borage decoction (preparation No. 35) at intervals of twenty minutes between each cupful.

Heath: massage with heath oil (preparation No. 39) the painful areas. Drink also a litre of heath decoction (preparation No. 38), taking it in several doses in the course of the day. Immersion in a heath bath is also recommended. Boil 500 g of heath in four litres of water for fifteen minutes. Strain and add the decoction to the water of a hot bath. Lie in the bath for twenty minutes.

Camomile: massage the painful areas with camomile oil (preparation No. 43).

Ash: for three consecutive weeks drink before breakfast a cup of ash leaf decoction (preparation No. 83) and another cup before retiring at night.

Nettles: drink a cup of stinging nettle decoction (preparation No. 123) one hour after each of the three main meals.

Parsley: put in a saucepan five tablespoonfuls of coarsely chopped parsley to a litre of cold water; bring slowly to the boil, allow to boil for five minutes and leave to infuse for fifteen minutes.

Drink a large cupful of the preparation before the midday and evening meals.
Meadowsweet: take a cup of meadowsweet infusion (preparation No. 137) before each of the three main meals.
Willow: put in a saucepan one and a half tablespoonfuls of willow bark to half a litre of cold water; bring slowly to the boil, boil for ten minutes and strain. Drink this liquid before the midday meal and before the evening meal in two equal doses.

SCIATICA

Nettle massage

According to popular medicine the most efficacious method of combating sciatica is to beat the painful areas with stinging nettles, remembering to carry out the procedure with a light hand. When the skin has reddened use white wine on it as a lotion.

Clematis alcohol

Dab the painful area three times a day with a piece of cotton wool soaked with alcohol of clematis (preparation No. 62).

Egg white poultice

Beat some egg whites to a stiff consistency. Spread on a piece of thick water-resistant cloth. Sprinkle the egg white with ground pepper and apply to the affected areas.

Walnut husk poultice

Chop finely some of the husks of walnuts (in fact the fleshy fruit that surrounds the actual nut) and enclose them in gauze which is then applied to the painful areas.

Cabbage poultice

Melt in a *bain marie* some lard and dip into it some cabbage leaves which are then applied to the painful spots as hot as is bearable by the patient. Cover with a flannel and leave the poultice in place until it is cold.

STIFF NECK

Rosemary method

Chop two large twigs of rosemary. If the herb is not available fresh use an adequate amount of dried rosemary. Place in a saucepan the chopped twigs or dried herb, as the case may be, together with half a litre of red wine; bring slowly to the boil and let it simmer for ten minutes. With a skimmer remove the rosemary which is then wrapped in a piece of gauze long enough to go around the neck. Cover with a double thickness of dry flannel which in turn is covered with a woollen scarf. Maintain the poultice in place as long as it remains warm.

Thyme method

Chop a generous amount of fresh thyme and put it, by itself, into a frying-pan or saucepan. While it is heating turn it constantly and remove from the heat when it begins to frizzle. Wrap the thyme in a piece of gauze of an adequate length and wrap around the neck. Cover the poultice with a woollen scarf and leave in place until the poultice is no longer warm.

First-aid method

If no rosemary or thyme is available the pain can be alleviated by winding around the neck a strip of gauze containing laurel leaves which have been heated and prepared in the same manner as the thyme above. If laurel is not available rub the neck with a pad of cotton wool soaked with olive oil, covering the neck afterwards with a woollen scarf.

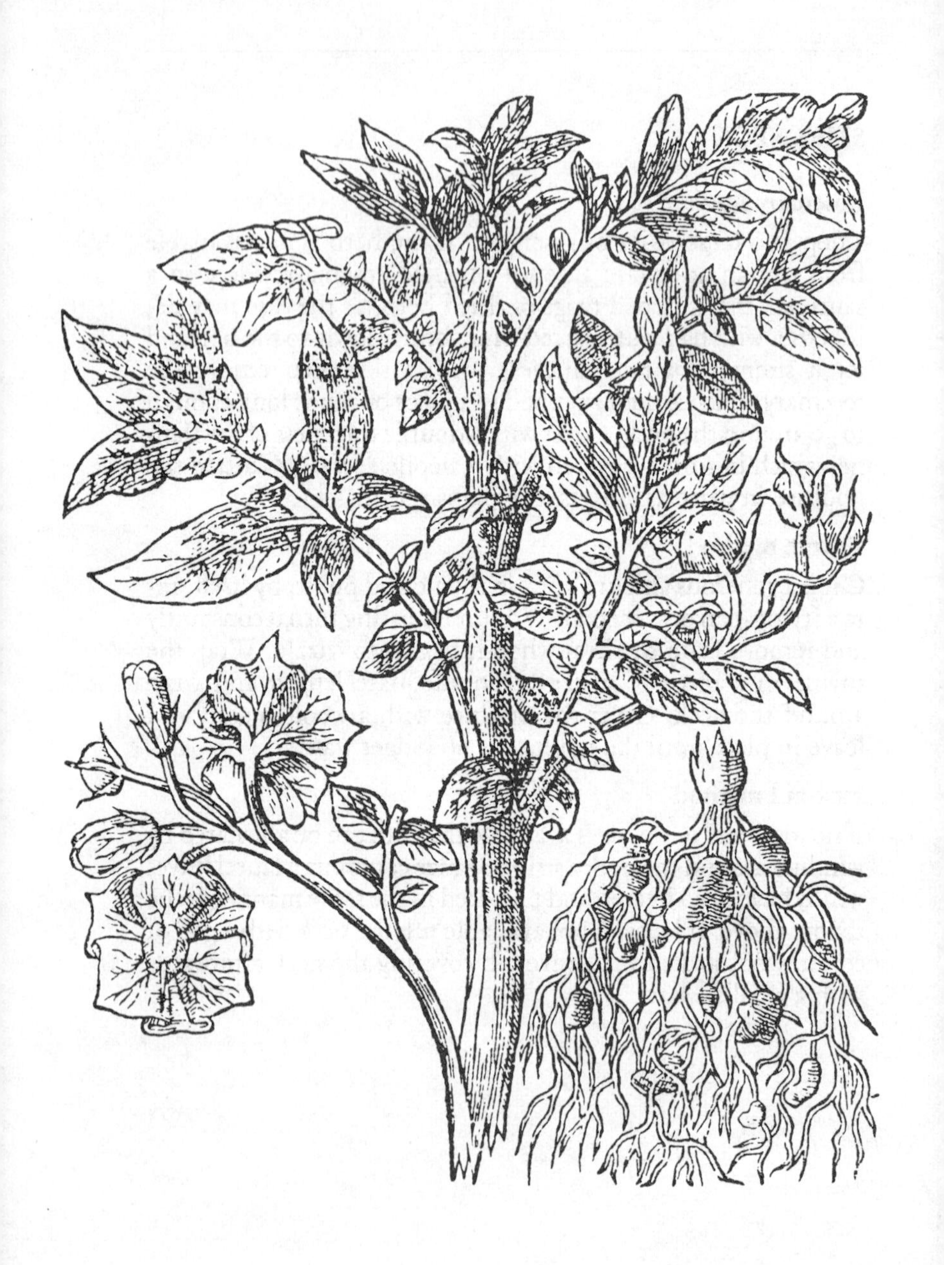

The Skeleton

DECALCIFICATION · FRACTURES · RICKETS
SPINAL CURVATURE

DECALCIFICATION

Horsetail infusion

Take a cup of horsetail infusion (preparation No. 131) first thing in the morning and last thing at night for a period of three weeks.

Eggshell method

Crush thoroughly an eggshell and place it in a bottle that can be hermetically sealed; add the juice of a lemon, cork, shake the bottle well and leave in a cool place for two hours. Then top up the preparation with half a litre of still mineral water and a few lumps of sugar. Shake well again and strain. Drink the decoction several times a day and follow the treatment for three weeks.

FRACTURES

In all popular medicine methods suggested for the reduction of fractures there is a risk of the patient being crippled for life. Call a doctor immediately to attend to a fracture and until his arrival place the fractured limb on a hard, flat surface, filling any space between the limb and the surface with cotton wool so that it rests totally immobilized.

RICKETS

Sunbathing, the more of it the better, is recommended by popular medicine as a method of fighting rickets. Sleeping on a mattress filled with birch leaves is also advised. The leaves must first have been dried in an oven.

In some regions of France the following mixture is preferred to birch leaves: oat straw, elder flowers, camomile flowers, melilot flowers, ferns, sprigs of mint in flower, sage and sweet marjoram. If some of these plants are not available mix together those of them that you can find, dry them thoroughly and fill your mattress with them.

There is also a recommendation to take either an aperitif glass of watercress wine (preparation No. 67) before each of the three main meals or a small liquor glass of rose hip syrup after the midday and evening meals (preparation No. 73).

SPINAL CURVATURE

Pine lotion

Put into a saucepan 200 g of a mixture of pine and fir needles to a litre of cold water. Bring slowly to the boil and simmer for twenty minutes, strain through a cloth, squeezing well. Add to the liquid 100 g of alcohol at 90° and store in a bottle. Rub every night the back, shoulders and trunk with the preparation.

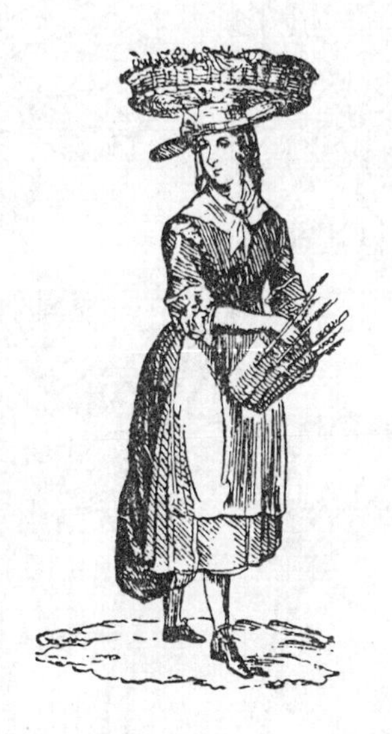

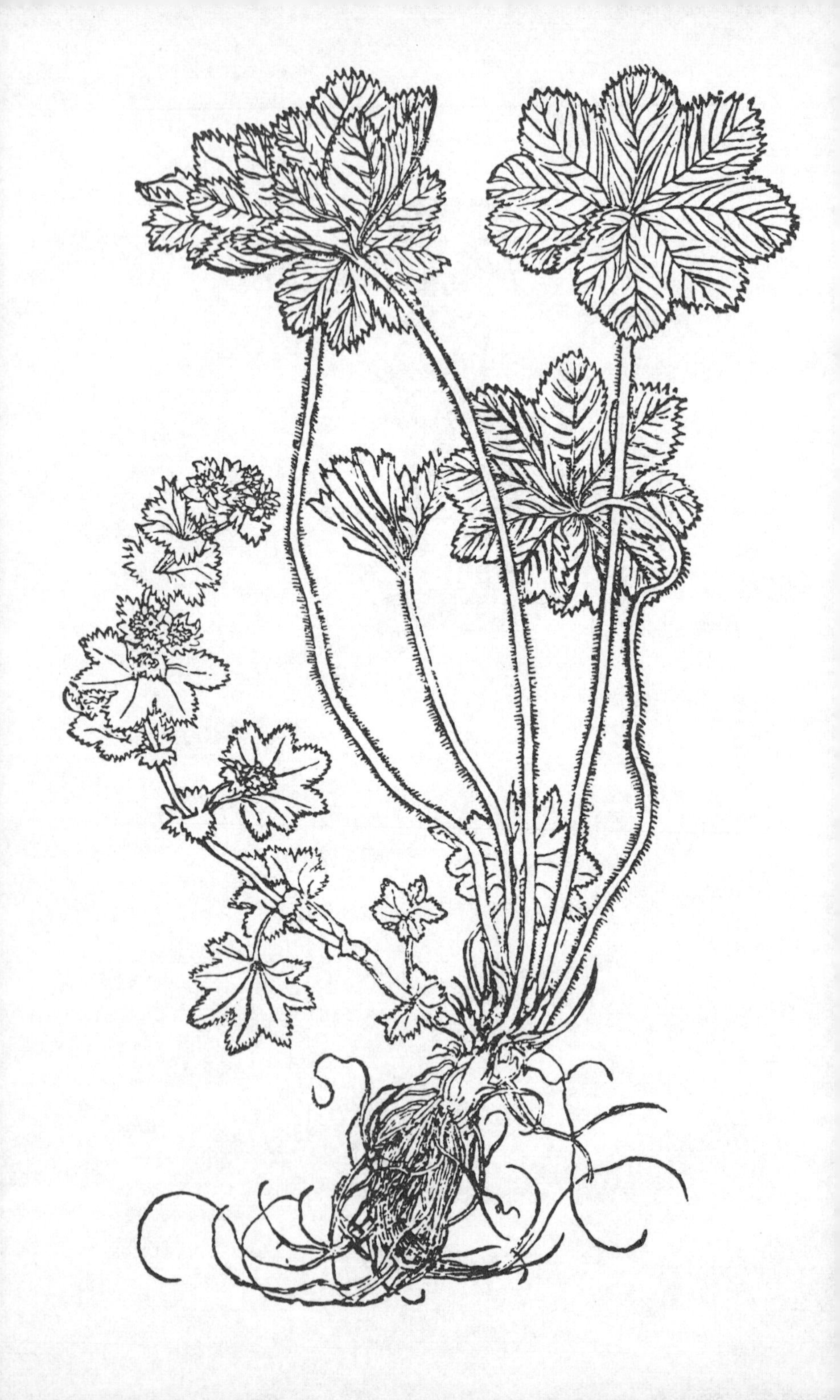

Skin and Hair

SKIN DISEASES · ITCHING · ACNE
BLOTCHINESS OF THE FACE · DARTRES (SCABBING)
ECZEMA · ERYSIPELAS · SCABIES · HERPES · IMPETIGO
LUPUS · BLACKHEADS · PSORIASIS · RINGWORM
URTICARIA (NETTLERASH) · SHINGLES · TO FADE FRECKLES
CARE OF GREASY SKIN · CARE OF DRY SKIN
TO CLEAR THE COMPLEXION · ALOPECIA (BALDNESS)
TO CHECK FALLING HAIR

SKIN DISEASES

Folk medicine has handed down to us a collection of methods for use in cases of skin afflictions but without being specific as to what these 'afflictions' comprise. One can therefore fall back on these methods in the treatment of a skin condition for which no specific remedies have been given or when others have proved to have no effect.

In general, for skin complaints folk medicine recommends:

(1) Follow a diet of uncooked vegetables and fruit and fresh vegetable and fruit juices for one day in each week.

(2) Apply as a lotion to the affected areas either olive oil, walnut oil or cabbage juice.

Sundry methods

Persicaria: collect before sunrise some persicaria (lady's thumb) and rub it on the affected parts while the dew is still fresh on it.
Dandelion: take a cupful of dandelion infusion (preparation No. 129) a quarter of an hour before each of the principal meals. If the infusion has no effect try the dandelion decoction (preparation No. 128) taken in similar doses at the same times.
Salsify: put into a saucepan six tablespoonfuls of chopped salsify roots to a litre of cold water. Bring slowly to the boil and keep it boiling for half an hour then strain. Take a cupful of decoction first thing in the morning, another between breakfast-time and

the midday meal and a third between the midday and evening meals.
Soapwort: dab the affected areas with soapwort decoction (preparation No. 142).
Scabious: put in a saucepan a coffeespoonful of dried root of field scabious to half a litre of cold water. Bring slowly to the boil, boil for half an hour, leave to infuse for fifteen minutes and strain; take in the morning, on an empty stomach, two coffee-cupfuls of the decoction.
Marigold: dab the affected parts three times a day with a lotion of marigold infusion (preparation No. 150).
Violets: take a cup of violet decoction (preparation No. 167) before each of the main meals. Also, twice a day, dab the affected areas with the same preparation.

ITCHING

The undermentioned methods may be used where a skin affliction is accompanied by itching. When, therefore, one is in the dark as to the cause of the complaint one can resort to these methods, or use them to complement a specific treatment for a condition that has been recognized (e.g. urticaria (nettlerash) where the following methods may be used in addition to the specific popular medicine treatment, a fumitory bath).

Great care must of course be taken to avoid mistaking certain infectious diseases such as those, like measles for example, which are accompanied by skin eruptions, for skin diseases.

Cucumber juice

Cut thin slices from a cucumber that has first been peeled and place them in a salad bowl where they should remain for two hours.

Collect the juice by filtering it through a fine cloth, pressing and squeezing the slices thoroughly. Dab the affected areas with this liquid or apply compresses that have been soaked in it.

Sundry methods

Lady's mantle: rub the affected parts three times a day with a decoction of lady's mantle (preparation No. 4).
Camomile: rub the affected parts three times a day with an infusion of camomile (preparation No. 45).
Bittersweet: either rub the affected areas with bittersweet lotion (preparation No. 71) or apply compresses soaked in it. Treat three times a day by either method.

ACNE

Diet

According to popular medicine those who suffer from acne should eat raw vegetables and fresh fruit as much as possible. Eating half a pound of dates every day and a raw turnip, which should be chewed thoroughly, is particularly recommended.

Sundry methods

Burdock: wipe the pimples with a piece of cotton wool soaked in burdock decoction (preparation No. 21).
Lettuce: use a decoction of lettuce (preparation No. 93) and proceed as for burdock.
Lavender: use an infusion of lavender (preparation No. 94) and proceed as above.
Nettles: put in a saucepan three tablespoonfuls of stinging nettle leaves to half a litre of cold water; bring slowly to the boil and keep on the boil for ten minutes before straining. Apply to the spots compresses soaked with this decoction.
Tomato: in the evening, before going to bed, rub the spots with slices of tomato. Allow to dry for half an hour and then wash off with cold water. The following day proceed in the same way at the same time but substituting crumpled sorrel leaves for the tomato. On the third evening apply tomato again, on the fourth sorrel, and so on, alternating the treatments until the condition has improved.

BLOTCHINESS

Horse Chestnut method

Remove the outer, prickly part of four large horse chestnuts and cut the 'conkers' into small pieces. Put the horse chestnuts in a saucepan with a litre of cold water. Bring slowly to the boil, allow to boil for a quarter of an hour then strain.

Dip a piece of cotton wool in the lotion and wipe it over the face morning and night.

Sundry methods

Lavender: apply to the face a lavender infusion (preparation No. 95) morning and night.
Lime (linden): put in a receptacle two tablespoonfuls of lime tree (linden) flowers; pour on half a litre of boiling water; stir well and cover; leave to infuse for ten minutes before straining. Massage thoroughly the face morning and evening with the infusion.
Vine leaves: rub the face morning and evening with a piece of cotton wool soaked in a decoction of vine leaves (preparation No. 166).
Footbath: according to popular medicine blotchiness of the complexion can be reduced by taking a warm footbath every morning.

DARTRES (SCABBING)

Calves' crow lotion

Place in a saucepan a kilo of chopped calves' crow (mesentery) with three litres of water. Bring to the boil, simmer for an hour and allow the broth to cool a little before being strained through a fine cloth.

Heat the liquid before use and wash the scabs thoroughly morning and night. Dry with a soft cloth.

Walnut ointment

Pound in a mortar 50 g of walnut with an equal amount of salt and add, little by little, a coffeespoonful of vinegar until a smooth paste is obtained. Apply the ointment to the scabs at night.

Another method is to apply direct to the scabs the juice extracted from fresh walnuts.

Sugared vinegar

Dissolve some Demerara sugar in wine vinegar until the liquid has reached saturation point. Rub the affected spots with the preparation morning and night.

Sundry methods

Burdock: dab the scabs with a decoction of burdock root (preparation No. 21) morning and night.

Mullein: put in a saucepan two teacupfuls of mullein flowers and leaves to a litre of boiling water; boil for ten minutes and strain. Apply to the dartres compresses soaked in the solution.

Another method is to apply fresh mullein leaves to the scabs.

Alder buckthorn: mix in a container a litre of alder buckthorn decoction (preparation No. 34) with a litre of wine vinegar and a litre of boiled water. Wash the flaking skin twice a day with the preparation which should always be heated, but not to boiling point, before being used.

Carrots: apply compresses of grated carrots to the dartres.

Greater Celandine: extract the juice from fresh greater celandine leaves and apply to the dartres.

(Translator's note: be sure that the leaves of the Greater Celandine *(Chelidonium majus)* are used and not those of the Lesser Celandine *(Ranunculus ficaria)* for which this particular healing property is not claimed. More important, take care that the juice is applied only to the affected patches as it can produce sores on healthy skin – as was well-known to medieval beggars seeking sympathy and alms.)

Cabbage: before going to bed apply some cabbage leaves to the dartres, keeping them in place with a bandage throughout the night.

Lemon: mix 100 g of soft butter with the juice of two lemons. Apply the ointment to the skin at night.

Bittersweet: wash the affected parts morning and evening with a lotion made from bittersweet (preparation No. 71).
Holly: boil some fresh holly leaves in a small amount of water. Replace the water when necessary as it boils away. When the leaves are thoroughly cooked chop them and apply them to the dartres.
Scarlet pimpernel: apply to the affected areas some fresh scarlet pimpernel leaves which have been lightly pressed with a warm iron.
Elm: apply at night some elm ointment (preparation No. 122) and massage in the morning with elm decoction (preparation No. 121).
Soapwort: use a decoction of soapwort (preparation No. 142) as a lotion morning and night.
Sage: crush with a rolling pin or bottle fresh sage leaves and apply to the affected areas.
Salt: dissolve in a glass of water a tablespoonful of rock salt and apply to the dartres compresses soaked in this preparation.
Veronica: moisten the dartres with a pad soaked with a warm decoction of veronica (preparation No. 161).

ECZEMA

According to popular medicine those afflicted with eczema could alleviate the condition considerably if they were to eat each day two raw carrots and a small raw turnip, chewing thoroughly.

Oil of lavender

Put in a receptacle five tablespoonfuls of lavender flowers to half a litre of olive oil. Heat in a *bain marie* for two hours, after which leave to macerate during the night. On the next day, strain through a cloth, taking care to squeeze the lavender flowers as you do so.

Apply each night the oily lotion to the affected areas.

Quince leaf poultice

Melt in a frying-pan a piece of fresh pork fat, complete with rind.

Toss into the hot grease some quince leaves and remove the pan from the heat at once.

Apply the greased leaves to the skin in need of treatment and cover with gauze and a dressing and keep the poultice in place for at least two hours.

Burdock poultice

Toss into some boiling milk some burdock leaves; simmer for five minutes before removing the leaves. Apply them to the affected areas, cover with gauze and keep the poultice in place for at least two hours.

Sundry methods

Box: apply three times a day to the affected areas a lotion made of a decoction of box leaves (preparation No. 41). At the same time, and for a period of one week, drink four cups daily of the same decoction: one in the morning on an empty stomach, one in the middle of the morning and one in the middle of the afternoon, and the fourth on retiring.

Calvados: put into half a litre of calvados 2 g of salicylic acid. Apply this liquid as a lotion twice a day to the affected areas.

Camomile bath: put in a large receptacle ten tablespoonfuls of camomile flowers to four litres of cold water. Bring slowly to the boil and keep it on the boil for ten minutes, then leave to infuse for five minutes. Strain and pour the decoction obtained into the bath water in which the patient should soak until the water cools.

Greater celandine: apply to the affected areas some greater celandine ointment (preparation No. 54) every night. *(Translator's note:* see the warning p. 67)

Oak bark: apply to the affected areas the lotion made from oak bark decoction (preparation No. 58) twice daily.

Bittersweet: take each morning on an empty stomach a cup of bittersweet decoction (preparation No. 69). At the same time apply the decoction to the affected areas every night.

Bilberry: twice a day apply to the affected areas some lotion made from bilberries (preparation No. 112). *(Translator's note:* the bilberry *Vaccinium myrtillus)* is called *myrtille* in French and goes under many names in Great Britain including whortleberry, blaeberry, whinberry, wimberry, hurtleberry, hurts, huckleberry, and in the Western Isles of Scotland the dried leaves were used as a substitute for tea. It should not be confused with the bog myrtle *(Myrica gale)* which belongs to a different botanical family.)

Nettles: put in a saucepan two tablespoonfuls of fresh leaves and stems of stinging nettles, chopped into small pieces, to a litre of cold water. Bring slowly to the boil and maintain at boiling point until the liquid is reduced to half the original volume. Strain and drink the liquid in several draughts in the course of the day.

ERYSIPELAS

White of egg poultice

Beat until stiff the white of an egg with a tablespoonful of vinegar. Apply to the affected areas in the form of compresses previously soaked in the mixture.

Dried bean poultice

Cook in salted boiling water some dry kidney beans and when thoroughly cooked mash them and wrap them in gauze cut to an appropriate size to cover the affected areas.

Lady's mantle

Soak in water for a short while some leaves of lady's mantle and apply them to the affected areas, ensuring that the upper surface of the leaves comes in contact with the skin.

Walnut emulsion

Beat hard some walnut oil with some water, in equal proportions of a coffeecup of each. Apply the emulsion to the affected areas three times a day.

SCABIES

(Translator's note: La gale is an old-fashioned French term for a variety of afflictions manifested by scabs and itching. Used in the figurative sense it is a term of derision or abuse similar to the use in English of 'scurvy knave', 'scab' etc. It is as medically imprecise in French as 'rash' is in English. If and when it is applied to scabies it should be remembered that this condition, which occurs most usually between the fingers, inner side of the wrist, on the buttocks and in the crotch, is caused by a parasitic mite, acurus, so care must be taken to avoid re-infestation by, for example, wearing gloves, socks and underclothes which have not been thoroughly cleaned.)

Bathing with burdock decoction
Mix a litre of burdock decoction (preparation No. 34) with a litre of lukewarm water and a litre of wine vinegar. Bathe the affected areas in this liquid at least three times a day. The preparation should be warmed up each time before use.

Celery
Crush in a mortar a generous handful of fresh celery leaves adding at the same time and little by little 100 g of salt and a large glass of vinegar. Strain through a linen cloth while squeezing the residue at the same time. Apply the lotion to the affected areas for as long as is required.

Garlic
Take a head of garlic and peel separately each part of it. Boil the cloves of garlic in a litre of water. Strain. Wash at least twice a day the affected areas with the liquid.

HERPES

Soapwort lotion
Twice a day apply to the affected areas a lukewarm lotion of soapwort infusion (preparation No. 143).

Bittersweet treatment

Apply bittersweet lotion (preparation No. 71) twice a day to the affected areas. Also take twice a day a coffeecupful of bittersweet infusion (preparation No. 70): one cup in the middle of the morning and another one in the afternoon.

IMPETIGO

Marigold compresses

Put in a saucepan four tablespoonfuls of marigold flowers to half a litre of cold water; bring slowly to the boil, allow to boil for a quarter of an hour then strain.

Apply to the affected areas some compresses soaked in this decoction which must be used while still very warm but not scalding. Renew the compresses three times a day.

Soapwort

Three times a day apply to the affected areas a lotion made of soapwort infusion which should be used lukewarm (preparation No. 143).

Oak bark

Apply to the affected areas compresses soaked in a lukewarm oak bark infusion (preparation No. 58). Renew the compresses every hour.

LUPUS

Greater celandine ointment

Apply to the affected areas twice a day or more frequently if necessary some greater celandine ointment (preparation No. 54).

BLACKHEADS

Mint alcohol lotion

At night apply to the blackheads a lotion made of a mixture of alcohol of mint and rose water (preparation No. 108).

Tomato method
Massage thoroughly at night with tomato juice each area where blackheads occur. Next morning proceed in the same way but substituting for sliced tomato some crumpled sorrel leaves.

Elder water
Massage the face after moistening the hands with elder water (preparation No. 152).

PSORIASIS

Scientific medicine has as yet found no cure for psoriasis so the popular medicine methods mentioned here may well be worth trying.

Salt water baths
Take three times a week a hot bath in which two kilos of rock salt have been dissolved.

Soot ointment
Collect some soot from a chimney where wood is burned. Mix the soot with olive oil and when a smooth mixture has been obtained knead in some lard so as to make an ointment. Apply at night this ointment to the psoriasis and cover with bandages to avoid soiling clothes and sheets.

Sundry methods

Bittersweet: firstly, dab on the psoriasis, morning and night, a pad soaked in a solution of bittersweet (preparation No. 71). Secondly, take a cup of bittersweet infusion on an empty stomach in the morning and again before retiring.
Walnut leaf: take four cups of walnut leaf infusion (preparation No. 115) one first thing in the morning, one cup in the middle of the morning, one in the middle of the afternoon and the last and fourth cup before retiring.
St John's wort: mix a coffeecupful of St John's wort oil (prepara-

tion No. 109) with two coffeecupfuls of linseed oil. Dab the affected areas each night with the preparation.

Elm: take four coffeecups daily of elm decoction (preparation No. 121), namely: one cup half an hour before the main meals and one last thing at night.

Also apply to the affected areas some elm ointment (preparation No. 122).

Nettles: take four cups each day of stinging nettle decoction (preparation No. 123), namely: one on an empty stomach in the morning, another in the middle of the morning, a third in the middle of the afternoon and the fourth before retiring.

Also apply to the affected areas, morning and night, this preparation on a pad of cotton wool.

TINIA (RINGWORM)

Watercress poultice

Heat with some lard in a frying-pan a bunch of watercress. When the cress is thoroughly reduced remove it from the pan, allow it to cool a little and then apply it to the head, keeping it in place with a dressing and covering it with a towel. The poultice should be retained all night and the hair shampooed the following morning.

URTICARIA (NETTLERASH)

Fumitory bath

A method that is considered by popular medicine as the most efficacious way of treating urticaria is the fumitory bath. Put in a large container six tumblerfuls of fumitory and the same quantity of wild pansy flowers; add five litres of cold water, bring to the boil, leave to boil for five minutes and strain. Pour the decoction obtained into the water of a very warm bath. Soak in the bath for half an hour and on emerging dry the body lightly and use 90° alcohol as a massage on the affected areas.

SHINGLES

Soapwort is considered in popular medicine to be the specific for shingles. It appears to have been effective in certain cases but swift results should not be expected.

Take before the three main meals a cupful of soapwort infusion (preparation No. 143). Use, morning and night, soapwort decoction as well (preparation No. 142), applying it as a lotion.

TO FADE FRECKLES

Watercress lotion

Extract the juice from a bunch of fresh watercress. *(Translator's note:* this is most easily done with an electric blender, of course, but, failing that, a hand lemon-squeezer or a wooden spoon and a fine-mesh strainer will do just as well but takes longer.)

Put the juice in a flask or bottle *(Translator's note:* a Kilner jar is fine for this), and add honey, equal in amount to that of the juice. Shake well.

Apply to the face a cotton wool pad soaked in the preparation morning and night. Leave to dry for half an hour and then wash in cold water.

Dandelion decoction

Put in a saucepan a glassful of dandelion flowers to a litre of cold water. Bring slowly to the boil, boil for half an hour, strain through a fine cloth, pressing the flowers well. Wash the face morning and evening with this preparation.

Milk of cucumber

Macerate for two hours half a cucumber, cut into slices, in a quarter of a litre of fresh milk. Use as a lotion for the face and wash in cold water after three quarters of an hour.

CARE OF GREASY SKIN

Cucumber water

Boil in a litre of water an unpeeled cucumber, cut into cubes, for fifteen minutes. Strain through a cloth, squeezing the pieces of cucumber. Wash the face night and morning with this preparation.

Lemon juice

Use pure lemon juice as a lotion, applying it with cotton wool every morning.

CARE OF DRY SKIN

Melon juice

Mix some melon juice in a bottle with equal amounts of distilled water and fresh milk. Shake the bottle briskly so that the mixture is thoroughly emulsified. Use as a lotion on the skin of the face each night and wash if off in the morning.

Fresh milk

Dab the face with fresh milk. Wash in cold water a few hours later or, if applied at night, the following morning.

TO CLEAR THE COMPLEXION

Parsley lotion

Boil some coarsely-chopped parsley in half a litre of water for quarter of an hour. Strain through a cloth, squeezing well. Wash the face daily, morning and evening, with this preparation for a week.

Lemon

One evening per week massage the face with a slice of lemon after having washed it thoroughly with soap and water.

ALOPECIA (BALDNESS)

According to popular medicine, nettle juice has the property of stimulating the growth of hair.

Pound in a mortar some fresh stinging nettle leaves, place them in a fine cloth and press well to extract all the juice. Massage the bald patches briskly and thoroughly with this juice every night.

TO CHECK FALLING HAIR

Massage with olive oil

Rub the hair thoroughly at night with olive oil and go to bed with the head wrapped in a towel. Next morning shampoo the hair with tepid water and Marseilles soap. Follow this method for ten consecutive days. It may be repeated every month. *(Translator's note: savon de Marseille* is a common French laundry and household soap. The nearest thing to it in Great Britain is a good yellow soap of the kind usually sold in a long bar. If that cannot be found, use an unscented toilet soap of the type marketed as 'simple soap'.)

Egg massage

Beat two fresh eggs with a fork, as though for an omelette, into half a litre of tepid water. Rub the hair well with this preparation and let it dry before retiring. Wash the hair the following morning with tepid water and a good plain soap. Follow the treatment every third day for two consecutive weeks. The treatment may be repeated after an interval of two weeks.

Parsley powder

Reduce to a fine powder some parsley seeds (this is most easily done with an electric mixer or coffee grinder). Rub the powder briskly into the hair and scalp and leave until the following morning when the hair is washed with tepid water and a good plain soap. Use the treatment three times, leaving an interval of two days between each treatment. If necessary renew the treatment a few months later.

Thyme lotion

Put in a saucepan a glassful of thyme with a litre of cold water.

Bring slowly to the boil and keep on the boil until the liquid is reduced to half its original volume. Strain. Rub the hair with this lotion every night for one week.

Box alcohol

Chop finely 50 g of fresh box leaves. Place them in a bottle and pour half a litre of alcohol at 50°. Leave to macerate for a week, shaking the bottle twice a day. Strain. Rub the hair with this lotion for eight consecutive days, night and morning.

Green Walnuts

About 100 g of young green walnuts are needed for this preparation. Cook them in a *bain marie* with 300 g of lard for half an hour. Crush thoroughly in a mortar until a smooth ointment is obtained. Massage the head with it every night for one week, shampooing the hair each morning.

Watercress juice

Mix equal amounts of watercress juice and 70° alcohol. Massage the head with this night and morning for one week.

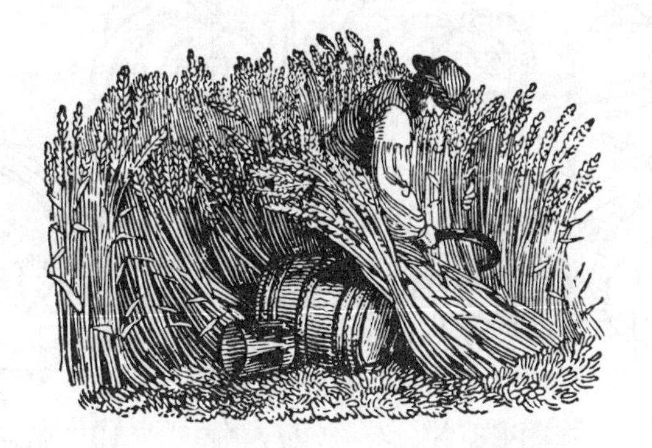

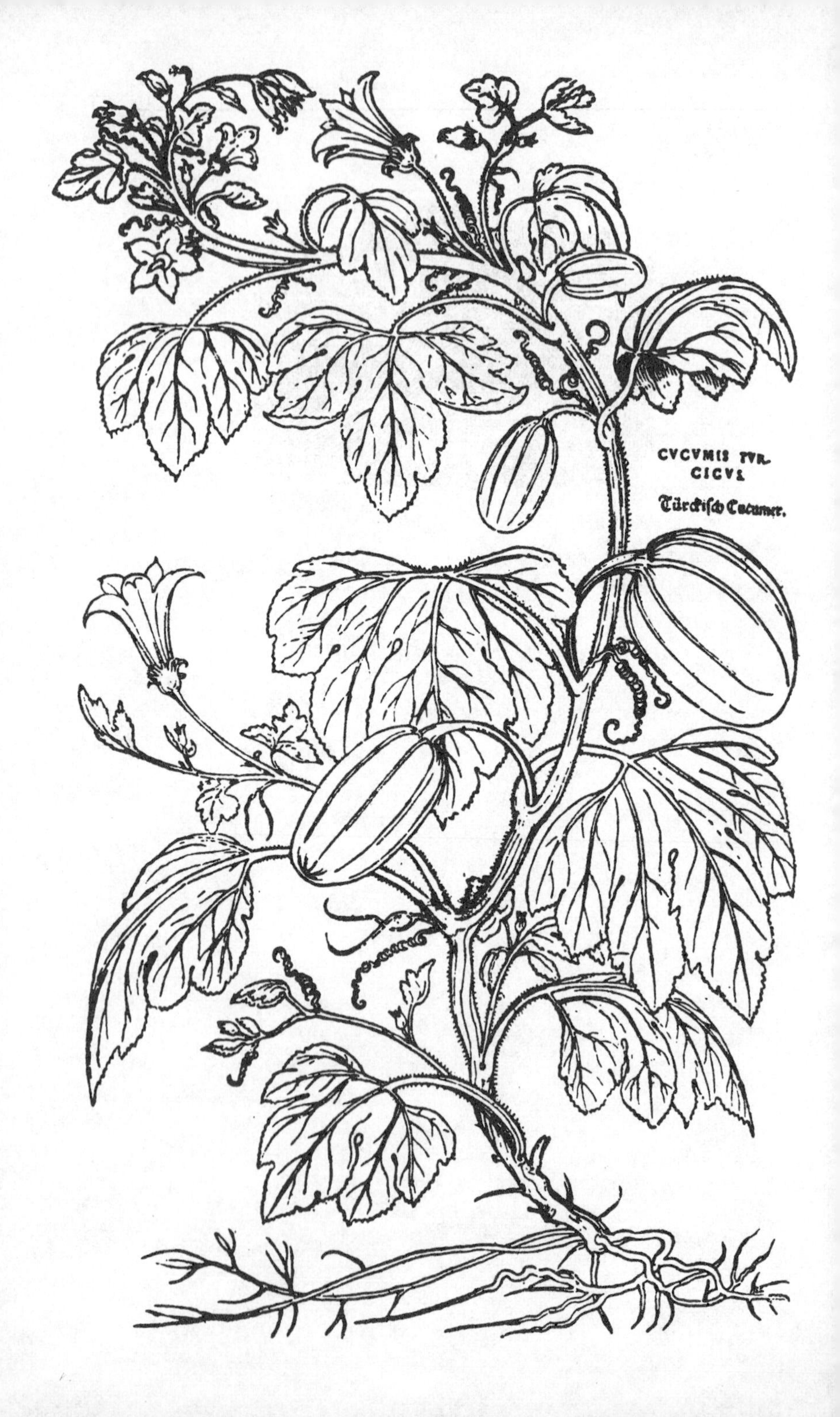
CVCVMIS TVR-
CICVS
Türckisch Cucumer.

The Respiratory Tract

DISEASES OF THE RESPIRATORY TRACT
TO SOOTHE A COUGH · TONSILITIS · ASTHMA
BRONCHITIS · HOARSENESS AND LOSS OF VOICE
SORE THROAT · INFLUENZA · COLDS

DISEASES OF THE RESPIRATORY TRACT

It is difficult to know what is meant in folk medicine by 'diseases of the respiratory tract'. What is implied is probably the respiratory distress that accompanies flu and colds. However, it is obvious that in cases where symptoms appear to be serious medical opinion should be sought.

Cabbage and leek poultice

Cook slowly in a frying-pan about a dozen cabbage leaves and two coarsely-chopped leeks together with a glass of vinegar. When the liquid is completely reduced enclose the preparation in a piece of gauze and apply it to the chest, covering it with a piece of flannel. Retain the poultice until it is cold. Another method is to apply to the chest some cabbage leaves that have been left in a hot oven for five minutes.

Sundry methods

Bittersweet: take a cup of bittersweet infusion after each of the three main meals (preparation No. 70).

Eucalyptus: take five cups of eucalyptus decoction in the course of the day, between meals (preparation No. 78).

Also inhale eucalyptus three times a day (preparation No. 79). Remember to cover the head with a towel so that none of the vapour rising from the inhalation cup escapes.

Thyme: take a cup of thyme infusion an hour before each of the main meals and another one just before retiring (preparation No. 156).

TO SOOTHE A COUGH

Horseradish syrup

Cut into rings some horseradish roots (if unavailable substitute large turnips). Place over a receptacle a colander and put into it a layer of horseradish (or turnip) slices covered with a layer of crystallized sugar. Make two more layers of horseradish and sugar and leave the preparation to macerate in a warm place for two or three hours. Collect the liquid and transfer into a bottle or jar. Take a tablespoonful of the syrup every hour or even more often if necessary.

Other methods

Gum arabic: melt 20 g of gum arabic in half a litre of hot water. Sweeten the preparation and take a few sips at the time of a coughing fit.
Greater celandine: take four cups of greater celandine infusion in the course of the day: a cup on any empty stomach in the morning, a cup in the middle of the morning and of the afternoon and the last one on retiring (preparation No. 54a).
Orange leaves: take at will small cupfuls of orange tree leaves (preparation No. 119).
Quince leaves: at the start of a coughing fit take a mouthful of quince leaf infusion (preparation No. 63).
Thyme: put in a saucepan a coffeecupful of thyme with half a litre of cold water. Bring slowly to the boil, boil for ten minutes and strain. Mix with the liquid 125 g of honey. Take a tablespoonful of this preparation at the onset of a coughing fit.

TONSILITIS

To fight tonsilitis popular medicine advises the use of various gargles and certain poultices. For a satisfying result one should apply both methods at the same time.

Laurel leaf poultice

Heat in a frying-pan an adequate amount of laurel leaves. Wrap up the leaves in a piece of gauze of an appropriate size to fit around the patient's neck; hold in place with a woollen scarf and maintain the poultice until it is cold.

Potato poultice

Prepare a very thick mash of boiled potatoes. Enclose the warm mash in a piece of gauze and wrap it around the neck, holding the poultice in place with a woollen scarf.

Leek poultice

Boil some leeks until they are thoroughly cooked. Strain, spread on a piece of gauze and sprinkle them with white pepper. Close the gauze, wrap around the throat and hold in place with a woollen scarf.

Garlic massage

Peel each piece of three heads of garlic and cook them slowly in 250 g of lard, gradually crushing them into it until an ointment is obtained. Rub this ointment thoroughly into the soles of the feet. After the treatment woollen socks should be worn.

Sundry methods

Lemon: pour into a glass the juice of a lemon. Fill the glass with boiling water and gargle with the preparation every two hours. After each gargle dab the pharynx with a cotton bud soaked in lemon juice.
Poppy: take in the course of the day four cups of infusion of poppy petals (preparation No. 65).
Oak bark: gargle with a warm decoction of oak bark three times a day (preparation No. 58) or with oak bark wine (preparation No. 59), which should be heated before use.
Blackcurrant: gargle several times during the day with a warm decoction of blackcurrant (preparation No. 48).
Turnips: boil slowly in a litre of water for half an hour 250 g of chopped turnips. Strain through a cloth, pressing well. Gargle with this preparation three times a day.
Liquorice: gargle four times a day with a maceration of liquorice (preparation No. 136). Also take every two hours a small cupful of liquorice decoction (preparation No. 134).

Sage: gargle at least four times a day with an infusion of sage (preparation No. 145).
Violets: gargle at least four times daily with violet decoction (preparation No. 167).
Apples: cook in a small amount of water some unpeeled apples (rennets for preference). When well cooked press well and strain through a cloth. Drink the preparation hot and sweetened to taste four times daily.

ASTHMA

Datura stramonium (thorn apple or jimson weed) cigarettes were the classic remedy for asthma in popular medicine. The leaves of the plant were dried and chopped as is done with tobacco leaves. But this plant is very toxic and cannot be bought. If one lives in a region where the plant can be found extreme caution should be observed and only two or three puffs of the cigarette should be taken. If relief is obtained a doctor should be consulted about further use. *(Translator's note:* this plant is not native to the U.K. but has become naturalized throughout England and Wales. It is a powerful hallucinogen and has various very potent pharmacological properties. As a remedy for asthma it should not be attempted lightly.)

Figs with eau de vie

Leave three dried figs to macerate during the night in *eau de vie*. Eat the figs before breakfast next morning.

Garlic alcohol

Place in a bottle three sliced cloves of garlic. Add a quarter of a litre of alcohol at 90° and leave to macerate for ten days, shaking the bottle twice a day. Strain and decant. During asthma attacks pour half a coffeespoonful of the preparation on a lump of sugar and let it dissolve slowly in the mouth.

Sundry methods

Angelica: put in a cup a generous tablespoonful of pieces of crystallized angelica. Fill the cup with boiling water, stir well and cover. Leave to infuse for ten minutes before straining. Take a cup of this infusion before each of the three main meals of the day.

Greater celandine: take for one month four cups per day of greater celandine infusion (preparation No. 54A): a cup on an empty stomach in the morning, one before each of the main meals and the last before retiring.

Poppy: during an asthma attack take a cup of infusion of poppy petals (preparation No. 65).

One can also prepare the following infusion: put in a receptacle a tablespoonful of poppy petals, a tablespoonful of eucalyptus leaves, a tablespoonful of ivy leaves, a coffeespoonful of violet flowers and two coffeespoonfuls of mullein flowers. Pour on three-quarters of a litre of boiling water, stir well, cover and leave to infuse for ten minutes. Strain. At the time of an asthma attack drink slowly a cup of this infusion.

Fennel: take before each of the three main meals a cup of fennel infusion (preparation No. 80).

Lavender: take four cupfuls per day of lavender infusion (preparation No. 94a): a cup first thing in the morning, one between meals and the last cup at least two hours after dinner and before retiring.

Mallow: at the time of asthma attacks prepare the following inhalation. Put in a receptacle two tablespoonfuls of mallow flowers and leaves and pour on a litre of boiling water, stir well and proceed to inhale, covering the head with a towel to concentrate the vapour.

Rosemary: put in a bottle five tablespoonfuls of rosemary, fill up the bottle with red wine and leave to macerate for a week, shaking the bottle twice a day. Strain and bottle. Take a small glass of this preparation during attacks. One can also take small mouthfuls of rosemary infusion (preparation No. 140).

Valerian: take before the three main meals a cup of valerian infusion (preparation No. 160).

Veronica: take five minutes before the three main meals a cup of unsweetened veronica infusion (preparation No. 162).

BRONCHITIS

Cabbage poultice

For the treatment of bronchitis popular medicine considers cabbage particularly efficacious.

Firstly, apply to the chest or to other areas, such as the back, where the pain is localized, a poultice made of several layers of cabbage leaves (preparation No. 55) and hold the poultice in place with flannel wrapped around the chest. One poultice to be applied during the day for at least four hours and another, on retiring, to be kept in place throughout the night.

Secondly, include in each of the principal meals a large plateful of cabbage soup and continue to do so for at least a week after recovery.

Milk-based preparations

1. Take twice a day, during the morning and during the afternoon, a bowl of cold milk to which has been added two large oysters. If the patient is put off by this unappetizing preparation try to swallow the oysters first and drink the milk immediately afterwards.

2. Take before retiring at night a well-sweetened bowl of hot milk to which has been added eight drops of tincture of iodine.

3. Boil slowly in a quarter of a litre of milk two chopped pieces of garlic. Allow to boil for fifteen minutes and then strain. Drink the preparation hot before retiring.

Horseradish poultice

Grate 250 g of horseradish roots and enclose them in a piece of gauze of suitable size. Apply the poultice to the chest and keep in place for a good hour.

Sundry methods

Cherry stalks: take during the course of the day a litre of cherry stalk decoction (preparation No. 52).

Poppy: take one hour after the three main meals a cup of infusion of poppy petals (preparation No. 65).

Watercress: take on an empty stomach in the morning and again

at night before retiring a coffeecupful of watercress juice. Also cook slowly in lard half a bunch of watercress, spread the preparation of a piece of gauze of an appropriate size and apply as a poultice to the chest, leaving it in place until it is cold.
Marsh mallow: take between meals three cups of marsh mallow infusion (preparation No. 88).
Orange leaves: take in the course of the day half a litre of orange leaf infusion (preparation No. 119).
Liquorice: take four cupfuls of liquorice decoction (preparation No. 134): a cup first thing in the morning, one between breakfast and the midday meal, another between the latter and the evening meal and the fourth on retiring.
Veronica: ten minutes before the main meals take a cup of unsweetened veronica infusion (preparation No. 162).
Violets: take five small cupfuls of violet decoction in the course of the day (preparation No. 167).

HOARSENESS AND LOSS OF VOICE

Decoction of celery

Put in a saucepan 100 g of chopped celery roots to a litre of cold water. Bring to the boil and boil slowly for three-quarters of an hour; strain while pressing firmly the celery and take the liquid obtained in several draughts throughout the day.

Agrimony gargles

Gargle three times a day with an agrimony infusion (preparation No. 1) into which two tablespoonfuls of honey to half a litre has been mixed.

Cabbage decoction

Put in a saucepan six large chopped cabbage leaves (preferably red cabbage) to a litre of cold water. Bring slowly to the boil, leave to boil for twenty minutes, strain through a fine cloth, taking care to press the leaves well. Drink this liquid during the course of the day.

Parsley infusion

Put in an infusion cup a finely chopped sprig of parsley and then fill the cup with boiling water. Cover and leave to infuse for six minutes before straining. Take four cupfuls per day of this preparation.

Hedge-mustard decoction

Take every two hours a cupful of hedge mustard decoction (preparation No. 149) hot and sweetened with a spoonful of honey. Drink the preparations in small mouthfuls, holding the liquid in the mouth before swallowing.

SORE THROAT

In addition to those methods recommended for tonsilitis, popular medicine has handed to us a number of remedies to cure any kind of sore throat without underlining precisely the type of ailment prevailing. Therefore, whenever a patient suffers from a sore throat the following remedies may be tried.

Hawthorn infusion

Put in a receptacle five tablespoonfuls of haws that have been dried and crushed. Pour on half a litre of boiling water, stir well, cover and leave to infuse for ten minutes before straining off the liquid.

Mix two tablespoonfuls of honey with the infusion and use as a gargle.

Sundry methods

Basil: gargle with an infusion of basil (preparation No. 22). Mix with it two tablespoonfuls of honey to half a litre of liquid.
Ewe's milk: gargle every three hours with hot ewe's milk.
Leeks: put in a saucepan four large sliced leeks to a litre of cold water. Bring slowly to the boil, boil for twenty minutes and strain. Pour the boiling decoction into a jug or other receptacle with a neck narrow enough to be covered with the wide opening of a funnel. Place the mouth over the funnel spout and breathe in the vapour.
Bramble leaves: place in a receptacle five tablespoonfuls of bramble leaves and pour on half a litre of boiling water, stir well,

cover and leave to infuse for ten minutes before straining. Add to the preparation a tablespoonful of peroxide of hydrogen and use the mixture as a gargle.
Thyme: chew slowly some sprigs of thyme several times a day.
Veronica: gargle three times a day with a warm decoction of veronica (preparation No. 161).

INFLUENZA

Influenza (or 'flu') is one of the few illnesses for which folk medicine can sometimes produce results as satisfactory as those brought about by orthodox medicine. It is important, however, to act as soon as the symptoms first appear.

Also one must not forget that certain types of influenza can be particularly serious and proper caution should be observed by calling a doctor if there is no quick and visible improvement in the patient's condition.

Guarding against influenza

When there is an epidemic the risk of contracting influenza may be lessened by taking a glass of cabbage juice before each of the two main meals of the day. The juice is obtained quickest with a blender but if one is not available cut the cabbage leaves into fine strips and rub through a sieve.

Drinks to be taken at the onset of influenza

The following is one of the most helpful drinks when it is felt that influenza is coming on. Collect the juice of an orange and lemon. Add to the juice two liqueur glasses of rum and six lumps of sugar. Heat without bringing to the boil and drink the preparation as hot as possible after getting into bed.

Another drink with a great reputation: boil gently a bowlful of good red wine to which has been added five lumps of sugar and half a grated nutmeg. Filter and drink hot.

Methods to apply at the onset of influenza symptoms

One should obviously try only one of the following methods at any one time but if there is no improvement on the following day a different one can be tried.

Footbath

Mix 100 g of mustard powder with very hot water. Bathe the feet in this preparation for a quarter of an hour, dry them and pull on some woollen socks before going to bed.

Inhalation and footbath combined

Fill a large receptacle, such as a cauldron or preserving pan, with boiling water and set it on a table. Sit at the table, cover your head with a towel and inhale the steam. At the same time place a bowl or basin half-filled with hot water under the table and soak your feet in it. Every three or four minutes replace some of the cooling water with hot water (it is obviously better if somebody can do this for you rather than interrupting both inhalation and footbath). After treatment wrap up warmly and go to bed.

Cold water method

The following procedure was renowned in the past. However, we have no record of just how effective it is, or if it could prove harmful. First put some hot water bottles in a bed specially made with a waterproof sheet. The patient is undressed and wrapped in a bath robe that has been soaked in cold water and well wrung out. He lies on the waterproof sheet with the hot bottles packed close to his body. These and the blankets in which he has been wrapped tightly should provide copious sweating. If after a few minutes a sensation of cold is still felt the treatment should be stopped at once. In any case it should not be prolonged beyond half an hour, after which the patient should be dried, dressed warmly and returned to a bed prepared in the normal way.

Hot water method

For this treatment some pieces of thick cloth, like old blankets, are required. They should be large enough for the patient to be wrapped in them from shoulders to waist, allowing for them to be crossed over in front like a large coat or cloak.

With the patient in bed close by, spread one of the pieces of cloth or blanket on a table. Soak another piece in boiling water, wring well and lay it on the dry cloth. Wrap up the patient's chest and back in the two cloths with the wet one next to the skin and the dry one on the outside. Cover the patient with blankets and prepare another set of cloths so as to carry out the treatment four times with an interval of five minutes between them.

Diet during influenza

During the first two days of an influenza attack folk medicine advises a diet of raw apples. A kilo, preferably grated, should be eaten in the course of the day. *(Translator's note:* the diet throughout influenza should, of course, be light and include plenty of fresh fruit.)

Drinks to be taken during influenza

The drinks listed below are said to hasten recovery from flu:

Basil: put in a saucepan two tablespoonfuls of basil to a litre of cold water; cover, bring slowly to the boil and boil for five minutes. Strain, add eight lumps of sugar and take small cupfuls of the decoction during the course of the day. It is to be taken cold.

Borage: take, preferably in the morning and at intervals of half an hour, four large cupfuls of borage decoction (preparation No. 35).

Box leaves: put in a saucepan five tablespoonfuls of dried box leaves to a litre of cold water; cover, bring slowly to the boil, boil for five minutes and leave to infuse for half an hour. Strain and take the decoction three or four times during the day. It should be drunk hot and well sweetened.

Camomile: take an infusion of camomile at the rate of three-quarters of a litre to be drunk per day (preparation No. 44).

Eucalyptus: take a decoction of eucalyptus in the quantity of three-quarters of a litre to be drunk in one day (preparation No. 78).

Lavender: drink between meals four cupfuls of lavender leaf infusion (preparation No. 95).

Elder: drink daily three-quarters of a litre of elder flower infusion (preparation No. 52).

Thyme: take after each of the three main meals a cup of thyme infusion (preparation No. 156).

Violets: take five cups per day of violet decoction (preparation No. 167).

Sundry methods

Onion: leave to macerate throughout the night two large thinly-sliced onions in half a litre of tepid water. Strain off the liquid next morning and take half before breakfast and the other half in the evening.
Eucalpytus: with whatever treatment is being used for influenza two eucalpytus inhalations daily must be combined with it (preparation No. 79). Remember to cover your head with a towel while inhaling.
Fennel: according to popular medicine recovery from influenza is hastened by chewing thoroughly some fennel seeds several times a day.

COLDS

Nutmeg method

Grate finely half a nutmeg. Place the grounds in a bottle; add a coffeecupful of *eau de vie* and half a coffeecupful of granulated sugar. Shake vigorously until it is well mixed.

Go to bed and drink the preparation in three or four mouthfuls. This method usually helps a lot but may produce nausea in some people.

Red cabbage syrup

Extract 250 g of liquid from a red cabbage. Mix the juice with 125 g of honey and two grams of saffron. Bring slowly to the boil, stirring all the time until a syrupy liquid is obtained.

Take a tablespoonful of this syrup four times a day mixed with one of the infusions listed later in this chapter.

Salt method

Use a rolling pin or bottle to reduce some table salt to a dusty powder. Place on your finger a small amount of this fine salt and sniff it, in the way in which snuff is taken, up one nostril while blocking the other with a finger. Then repeat with the other nostril.

This method usually produces good results but in some individuals may irritate the mucous membranes and should therefore be used with caution.

Onion method

Cut two pieces of onion to the size of small cloves of garlic. Wrap them in two separate strips of gauze and insert one into each nostril. Keep in place for five minutes while breathing deeply through the nose.

Lemon juice

Introduce into the nostrils a few drops of lemon juice several times a day.

Thyme method

This method is carried out in two steps:

First, put a tablespoonful of thyme in a cup which is then filled with boiling water. Cover, and allow to infuse for ten minutes. Strain and stir in a spoonful of honey. Take six cups per day of this preparation.

Also, place in a saucepan two tablespoonfuls of thyme to a cup of cold water. Bring to the boil, boil a for six minutes and strain.

Bend over the warm infusion and inhale the vapour through one nostril at a time, closing the other by pressing on it with a finger. Inhale deeply about ten times and repeat the treatment three times a day.

Other methods

Borage: take a generous cupful of borage decoction (preparation No. 35), warm and well sweetened, twice a day.

Poppy wine: place in a saucepan a tablespoonful of poppy petals, a level tablespoonful of borage flowers, a coffee-spoonful of lime flowers and half a litre of red wine. Bring slowly to the boil, boil for six minutes and strain. Take before retiring a large cup of the preparation which has been poured on to a few slices of lemon.

Holly: place in a receptacle about ten chopped holly leaves and pour on the equivalent of a large cupful of boiling water; stir

well, cover and leave to infuse for ten minutes before straining. Take the decoction on going to bed.
Marjoram: place in a receptacle a coffeespoonful of flowering marjoram and pour on a cupful of boiling water. Stir well, cover and leave to infuse for five minutes before straining. To a coffeespoonful of this preparation add a similar amount of glycerine. Place in each nostril a piece of cotton wool soaked with this liquid.
Turnip: place in a saucepan 100 g of chopped turnips to a litre of cold water; bring to the boil, boil for a quarter of an hour and strain. Take the decoction thus obtained several times in the course of the day.
Liquorice: take several cups a day of liquorice decoction (preparation No. 134) or liquorice maceration (preparation No. 136).
Tea: drink several times a day a cup of weak tea in which a coffeespoonful of sage has been infused.
Elder: as soon as the symptoms of a cold are felt take a cup of warm infusion of elder flowers (preparation No. 152); take another one an hour later and a third one before retiring.
Violets: take at will, except during the hour preceding main meals and the hour following them, a decoction of violets (preparation No. 167).

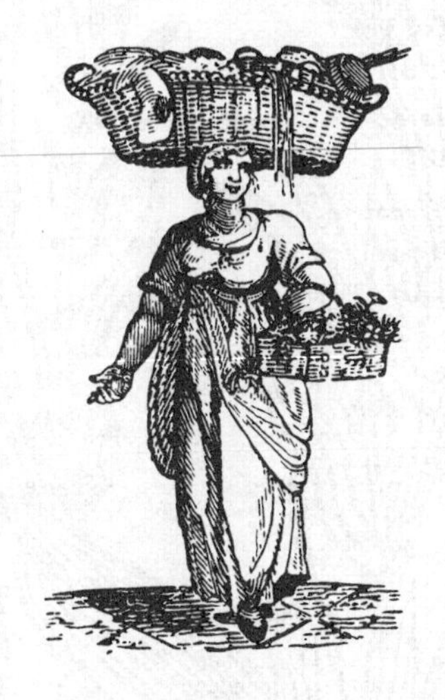

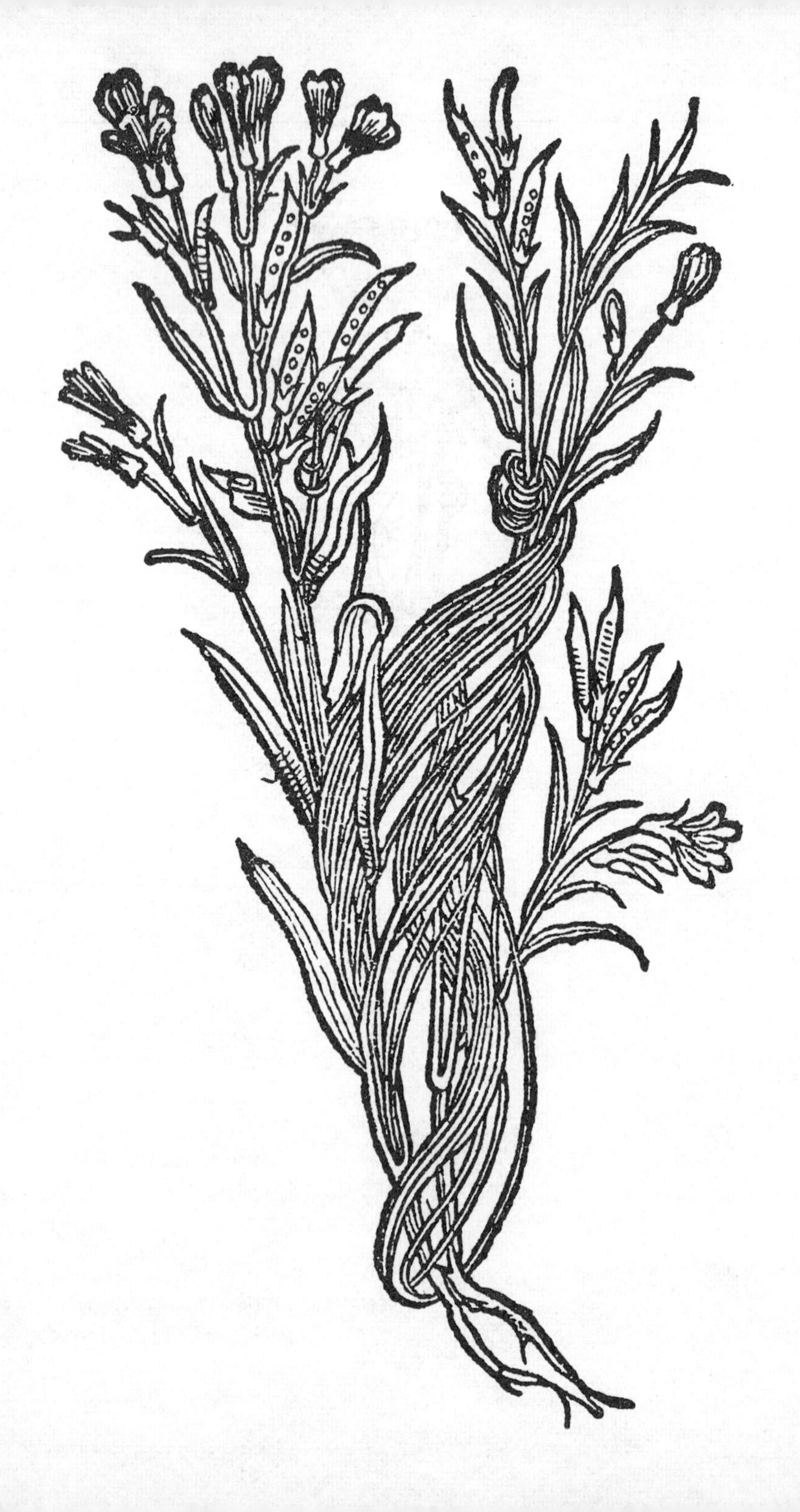

The Heart, Blood Vessels and Circulation

HEART DISEASES · ARTERIOSCLEROSIS · ARTERITIS
SWOLLEN LEGS · SWOLLEN HANDS · HAEMORRHOIDS
HIGH BLOOD PRESSURE · SYNCOPES
VARICOSE ULCERS · VARICOSE VEINS

HEART DISEASES

Whenever heart condition is mentioned in popular medicine it must be understood that it refers to minor conditions such as palpitation and not serious conditions such as angina and infarctus. We take it that anyone who has had a heart condition diagnosed is in regular touch with his doctor. But the methods listed hereunder may be considered as complementary to medical treatment.

Sundry methods

Asparagus: in cases of discomfort which may be due to the heart take at once a tablespoonful of asparagus syrup (preparation No. 18) and repeat for several days at the rate of one tablespoonful before the three main meals.
Hawthorn: take for ten days in the month before the main meals a cup of infusion of hawthorn flowers (preparation No. 19).
Dog rose: when feeling discomfort, drink a litre, taken in small cupfuls throughout the day, of rose hip decoction (preparation No. 72) and repeat for the three following days.
Broom: take before breakfast and last thing at night a large cupful of broom infusion (preparation No. 84).
Lettuce: when in discomfort take a cup of lettuce leaf decoction (preparation No. 93). Repeat for a few days, taking one cupful before retiring.
Mint: take first thing in the morning and before retiring a cup of mint infusion (preparation No. 106).
Lily-of-the-valley: take for one week in the month before lunch and dinner each day a cup of lily-of-the-valley infusion (preparation No. 111).

Onion: according to popular medicine heart sufferers should eat plenty of raw onions.
Parsley: take on an empty stomach first thing in the morning, and again before retiring, one cup of parsley infusion (preparation No. 126). Follow the treatment for one month.
Lime (linden): it is said that lime possesses properties to steady the heartbeat. Take a cup of lime decoction (preparation No. 138) before retiring.

ARTERIOSCLEROSIS

Diet

To combat arteriosclerosis folk medicine recommends taking every day between the two main meals the following: 50 g of sauerkraut, 100 g of raw watercress, a clove of garlic and a raw onion.

Wood avens (or Herb bennet) decoction

According to popular medicine wood avens is the specific for arteriosclerosis.

Prepare a decoction in the following way: place in a saucepan six tablespoonfuls of dried wood avens roots to a litre of cold water, leave to soak for an hour, bring slowly to the boil, cook for ten minutes and then remove from the heat. Allow the preparation to cool before straining.

Take one cup of the decoction after each of the three main meals.

Chervil infusion

Take before each of the three main meals one cup of chervil infusion (preparation No. 51).

Mistletoe wine

Take first thing in the morning an aperitif glass of mistletoe wine (preparation No. 87).

ARTERITIS

Generally speaking, it would seem unwise to rely on popular medicine for the treatment of an illness as serious as arteritis. However, orthodox medicine up to now has not proved very successful, being unable to bring appreciable relief or to prevent amputation sooner or later. That is why we take the unusual step of recommending partients not to accept blindly doctors' prescriptions without having first of all tried the cabbage leaf method which, even if it has no marked effect, cannot in any way aggravate the condition. Naturally this opinion is subject to the possible discovery of other methods of scientific treatment. The cabbage leaf method consists of applying to the legs three or four layers of cabbage leaves which have been prepared according to preparation No. 55. Maintain the poultice all night and keep it in place with a dressing that is not too tight. If there is pain during the night change the poultice for another made of fresh leaves. The effect that the method may have can only be judged after about ten days' treatment.

SWOLLEN LEGS

(Translator's note: any swelling of the legs not having an obvious cause – e.g. bruising – should be referred without delay to a doctor.)

Sage infusion

In the case of chronic swelling take for one week in the month two cups per day of sage infusion (preparation No. 145). A cup should be taken on an empty stomach in the morning and the second one after the midday meal.

Walnut bath

Prepare a walnut leaf decoction in the following way: place in a receptacle 600 g of walnut leaves to a litre of cold water; bring to the boil, leave to boil for ten minutes and strain. Add this preparation to the hot water of a bath and soak the legs in it for a quarter of an hour. The legs should afterwards by splashed or sprayed with cold water.

Poultices

Beat together (with an electric blender if possible) half a litre of olive oil, a large glass of cold water and one cup of vinegar. Apply to the legs several layers of folded cloth soaked in the emulsion.

SWOLLEN HANDS

Fill a basin with very hot water, of a temperature that can be borne by the hands for a few seconds. Soak the hands in the water for about ten seconds and then hold them under a cold tap for the same time. Repeat the hot and cold treatment ten times.

HAEMORRHOIDS (PILES)

Popular medicine suggests a good many methods for the treatment of haemorrhoids and has a useful part to play in alleviating the discomfort caused by this distressing complaint. The difficulty is in finding which method suits which patient. *(Translator's note:* any serious attacks of haemorrhoids, i.e. where profuse bleeding occurs, should be referred to a doctor.)

The burnt cork method

This method reduces considerably the duration of an attack of piles as well as relieving the pain.

Char thoroughly two corks. With a rolling pin or bottle crush the cindery residue to a fine powder. Beat the white of an egg until it is stiff and add to it the burnt cork together with a coffee-spoonful of almond oil. Spread the preparation on a cloth and apply the cloth to the haemorrhoids.

Bilberry method

Place in a saucepan ten generous tablespoonfuls of either fresh or dried bilberries to a litre of cold water. Bring slowly to the boil and leave to boil for half an hour. Strain, and press well the fruit while doing so, through a fine cloth. Soak compress with this liquid and apply to the haemorrhoids. Every half an hour renew with another warm compress and proceed until there is a marked relief.

One can also use the decoction an an enema and the liquid should be held in the rectum for as long as possible. It must not be forgotten that the temperature of the enema should not exceed body temperature.

Horsechestnut method

This cure is composed of three stages:

1. Take one hour before the two principal meals a cup of horsechestnut decoction (preparation No. 100).
2. Take a hip bath to the warm water of which has been added a concentrated decoction of horsechestnut (preparation No. 101). Take the bath three times a day.
3. After each hip bath apply to the haemorrhoids a poultice of crushed horsechestnut mixed with almond oil.

According to folk medicine, to lessen the frequency of haemorrhoid attacks a small bag of chopped horsechestnuts should always be carried on the person.

Leek method

Chop twelve large leeks. Place them in a cauldron with eight litres of cold water, bring to the boil and boil until well cooked. Pressing the leeks well, strain through a fine cloth and use the decoction as a hip bath taken twice a day for half an hour each time. The liquid should be as hot as can be borne.

Onion method

Chop finely two large onions. Mix in enough butter to produce an ointment which is then spread on a cloth which is applied to the haemorrhoids.

Potato method

Grate as finely as possible some peeled potatoes which are then wrapped in a piece of gauze to make a poultice that can be applied to the haemorrhoids.

Soot method

Collect soot from a chimney where wood is burned. Only a small amount is needed and to it add the same quantity of the yolk of hard-boiled egg. Spread the mixture on a cloth and apply to the haemorrhoids.

Milk method

Mix equal quantities of fresh milk and *eau de vie*. Soak a compress with the preparation and apply to the haemorrhoids. When the compress is dry substitute a fresh one. Continue the treatment until a significant relief has been obtained.

Sundry methods

Mullein: apply to the haemorrhoids fresh mullein leaves which have been lightly crushed with a rolling pin or bottle.

Shepherd's purse: the following method may be employed to maintain the healthy state resulting from a cure. Place in a saucepan the stems and dried flowers of shepherd's purse in the proportion of five tablespoonfuls to a litre of cold water. Macerate for an hour, bring to the boil, boil for one minute, infuse for a quarter of an hour and strain. Take for three weeks one cup of this decoction before each of the main meals.

The following method is prescribed in case of bleeding: take every three hours a spoonful of shepherd's purse wine (preparation No. 36a) and also apply to the haemorrhoids compresses soaked in the wine.

Camomile: this method usually helps to relieve the pain of an attack. Place in a toilet pail (a plastic bucket will do just as well) two generous handfuls of camomile; pour on four litres of boiling water. Sit on the bucket so that the haemorrhoids are exposed to the steam.

Chervil: boil a large handful of chopped chervil with three litres of milk. Strain and use the decoction in a hip bath. Save the chervil and use it in a poultice to be applied afterwards to the haemorrhoids.

Cabbage: apply to the haemorrhoids several layers of cabbage leaves (preparation No. 55).

Bittersweet: this method is used only in cases where the haemor-

rhoids remain unbroken, i.e. do not bleed. Soak a compress in a hot lotion of bittersweet (preparation No. 71). While the compress is still warm apply it to the haemorrhoids and when it is cold apply a fresh compress and repeat the procedure until relief has been obtained.
Horsetail: take for twenty minutes three times a day a hip bath of horsetail decoction (preparation No. 130).
Willow: scrape with a knife the bark from young willow boughs. Apply the bark to the piles.
Tansy: use an infusion of tansy, as hot as possible, to be used in a hip bath for half an hour twice a day (preparation No. 153).
Vine: drink a cupful of wine decoction after each of the three main meals (preparation No. 166).
Retracting the haemorrhoids
Quite apart from the chosen treatment, a lasting relief can only be obtained if the haemorrhoids are retracted after having protruded during the effort of a bowel movement. Using gentle but firm pressure by the index and second fingers push the piles up into the anus. Naturally, the hands should be scrubbed thoroughly both before and after doing this.

HIGH BLOOD PRESSURE

Olive leaf infusion

According to popular medicine the leaves of an olive tree, taken in an infusion, have the ability to lower high blood pressure.

Take an infusion (preparation No. 118) three times a day: a cup first thing in the morning, a cup before lunch and one before supper. Drink the infusion at these times each day until a satisfactory result is noticed and then continue the treatment during one week in each month.

One may also prepare the following decoction: place in a saucepan twenty olive leaves to a bowl of cold water; cover, bring slowly to the boil and continue to let it boil slowly until half the liquid has evaporated. Strain. Drink this infusion hot and sweetened: a cupful on an empty stomach in the morning and another before retiring. Follow this treatment for a fortnight, leave an interval of a week and repeat until a satisfactory result is noticed. After that, as a precautionary measure, repeat the treatment for a few days each month.

Bathing the arms

The following method is said to contribute to the lowering of high blood pressure. A bath thermometer is essential: the water should be, to start with, at 34° C.

Put the arms in the water, resting the elbows on the bottom of the bowl. After ten minutes pour away part of the water until the temperature reaches 37° C. Then, ten minutes after that, raise the temperature to 40° C. Ten minutes after that, to 43° C. Finally, after a further ten minutes, dry the arms and put on a warm cardigan or long-sleeved pullover.

Take one bath like this in the morning and another in the evening. It is said that there is a swift improvement in the patient's condition in a comparatively short time..

Sundry methods

Garlic: once a week use a peeled clove of garlic as a suppository and try to retain it in the rectum throughout the night.

Hawthorn: take before each of the three main meals a cup of hawthorn flower infusion (preparation No. 19): follow the treatment for three weeks, leave it off for one week then continue for one week and repeat in this alternating manner until an improvement is noticed.

A hawthorn tincture can also be taken in place of the infusion, (preparation No. 20): one coffeespoonful in a little water before the three main meals. Follow the cure for three weeks.

Chervil: take before the three main meals a cup of chervil infusion (preparation No. 51). Follow the treatment until the condition has improved. After an interval of a week renew the treatment.

Misletoe: place in a receptacle seven leaves of mistletoe growing on an apple tree. Pour on a cup of boiling water; cover, leave to infuse for five minutes and strain. Drink two cups in the day: one first thing in the morning and one before retiring.

Walnut leaves: take a cup of walnut leaf infusion (preparation No. 115) before the three meain meals.
Valerian: drink before the three main meals a cup of valerian infusion (preparation No. 160).

SYNCOPES (FAINTING)

In a case of fainting, popular medicine recommends the following procedure: the patient should lie flat on his back, his clothes are loosened and his face is dabbed gently with a cloth soaked with cold water. Massage with cold water the palms of the hands and the soles of the feet and place under the patient's nose a cup of strong vinegar or a slice of raw onion. When the patient has come round give him a little cold coffee with some *eau de vie* in it.

VARICOSE ULCERS

Agrimony compresses

Popular medicine considers agrimony as the specific for varicose ulcers.

Place in a saucepan 200 g of dried agrimony (a mixture of stems, leaves and flowers) to a litre of strong red wine. Bring slowly to the boil, boil for five minutes, leave to infuse for an hour and strain.

First wash the sores with this preparation and then apply compresses which have been soaked in it.

Walnut oil compresses

Place in a saucepan a glassful of walnut oil and the same amount of white wine. Boil slowly for a quarter of an hour. Apply to the sores compresses soaked in this preparation.

Cabbage leaves

Apply a poultice of cabbage leaves to the sores (preparation No. 55) which is held in place with a bandage for four hours. Renew the poultices until a satisfactory degree of healing has resulted.

Sundry methods

Ivy: cook for a quarter of an hour some ivy leaves in red wine. Apply to the sores the leaves which are held in place with a dressing and remain for at least three hours.

Quince leaves: soak for ten minutes in hot red wine some quince leaves and apply them to the sores as a poultice held in place by a dressing. Leave it there for three or four hours.

Saint John's wort: wash the sores with Saint John's wort oil (preparation No. 109).

Persicaria or lady's thumb: wash in cold water some freshly-gathered persicaria and apply it to the sores. Hold with a dressing in place for about twenty minutes. Use this treatment no more than twice in one day.

Apples: grate some apples and place in a dressing which is then applied to the sores.

VARICOSE VEINS

Garlic broth

Put in a teacup three cloves of grated garlic: fill with boiling water, cover and leave to macerate during the night. Drink this broth on an empty stomach next morning. Follow the treatment for one month and subsequently for one week in the month.

Pine needle lotion

Toss into a litre of boiling water a kilo of mixed pine and fir needles. Leave to boil for five minutes, press and strain well and bottle.

Each night, use a pad of cotton wool soaked in this preparation to dab lightly the varicose veins, taking care to apply the lotion in the direction towards and not away from the heart.

Sundry methods

Witch hazel: drink after midday and evening meals a cup of witch hazel infusion (preparation No. 90).

Melilot: take four cups of melilot infusion (preparation No. 103)

in the day: a cup first thing in the morning, one in the course of the afternoon and the last one before retiring.
Vine leaves: after each of the three main meals of the day drink a cup of vine leaf decoction (preparation No. 166).

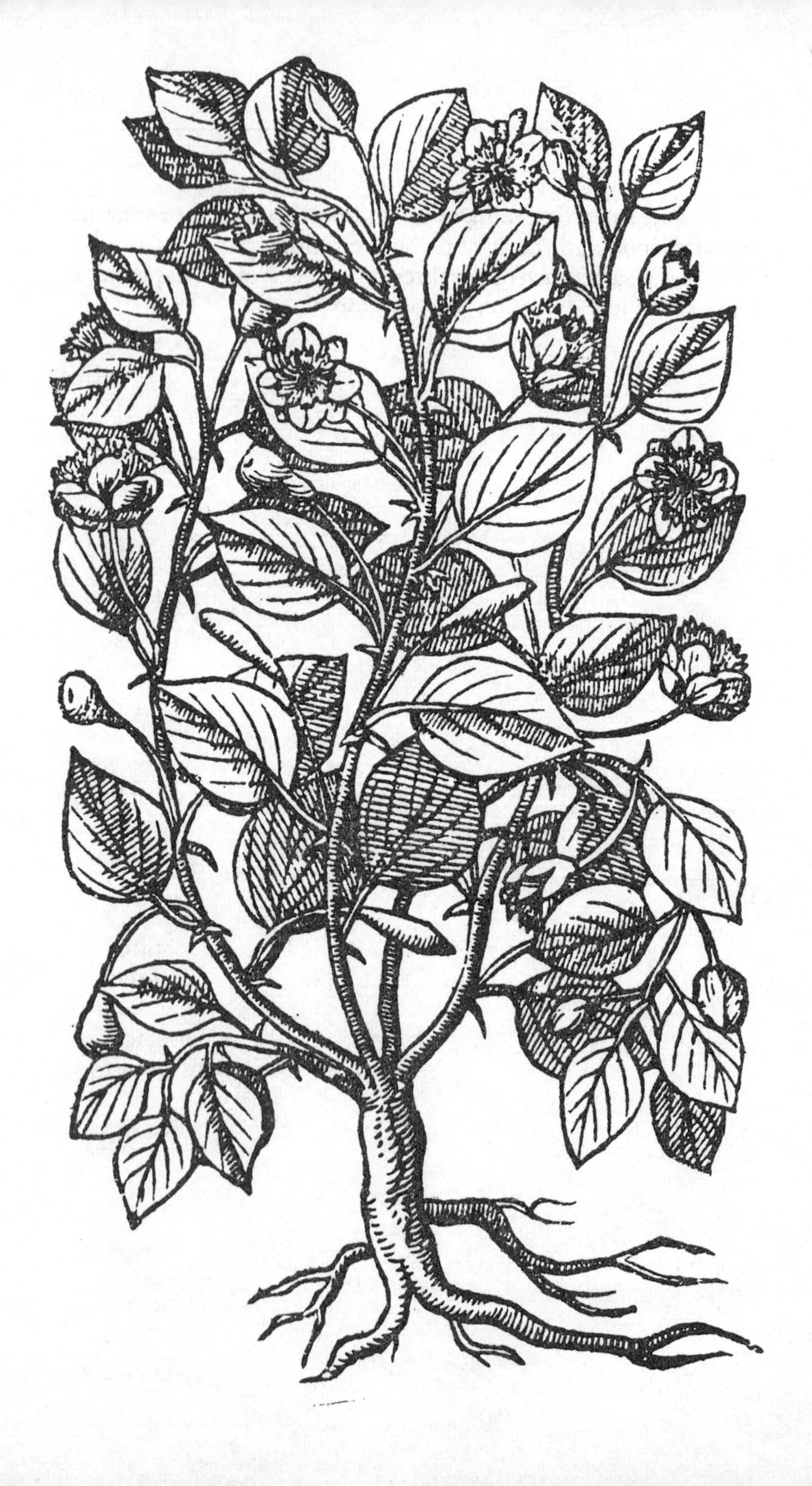

Food and Digestion

LACK OF APPETITE · AEROPHAGIA · COLICKY PAINS
CHRONIC ENTERITIS · CONSTIPATION
INTESTINAL DISORDERS · DIARRHOEA
STOMACH ACIDITY · DIFFICULT DIGESTION
STOMACH CRAMPS · STOMACH ACHE · STOMACH ULCERS
TO PREVENT INDIGESTION · INDIGESTION
LIVER DISORDERS · NAUSEA · INTESTINAL PARASITES
POISONING · DRUG ADDICTION · ALCOHOLIC
INTOXICATION · ALCOHOLISM · SCURVY

LACK OF APPETITE

Gentian wine

According to popular medicine gentian is supposed to be very efficacious in cases of anorexia where the patient's appetite needs to be stimulated. The following recipe is one that was often used in the past by country folk but the plant has become more difficult to obtain.

Place in a receptacle that has a lid three full tablespoonfuls of chopped root of yellow gentian and three coffeespoonfuls of centaury flowers; add a litre of 60° alcohol, cover and leave to macerate for two days, stirring three or four times a day. Pour a litre of white wine into this preparation, leave to macerate for ten days, stirring once a day, strain through a cloth, pressing well. Bottle.

Drink half an hour before midday and evening meals an aperitif glass of this wine.

Sundry methods

Thyme: chew slowly a small sprig of thyme an hour before each meal.

Sorrel: chop some sorrel leaves; place in a saucepan a tablespoonful of these to a cup of boiling water. Boil slowly for a quarter of

an hour, strain and drink the preparation three times during the day.
Camomile: take half an hour before the midday and evening meals an aperitif glass of camomile wine (preparation No. 46) or the infusion (preparation No. 44) if it is preferred to the wine.

AEROPHAGIA

Veronica infusion

According to popular medicine veronica is the specific for aerophagia. Take either the infusion (preparation No. 162) five minutes before each of the two main meals of the day or the decoction (preparation No. 161) half an hour before meals.

Sundry methods

Anis: take after the two main meals either a small liqueur glass of anis and cinnamon (preparation No. 11) or a cup of infusion of anis, caraway and cumin (preparation No. 12).
Tansy: take before each of the three main meals a cup of tansy infusion (preparation No. 12).

COLICKY PAINS

Colicky pains might be the sign of appendicitis. Therefore, if in any doubt, call a doctor before having recourse to one of the methods listed below. *(Translator's note:* such pains could also be the sign of food poisoning.)

Camomile syrup

In the past, to combat colic, camomile syrup was prepared in the following way.

Place in a receptacle 500 g of fresh camomile flowers; pour on three-quarters of a litre of boiling water, stir well, cover and leave to infuse for twenty-four hours. Squeeze well and strain through a cloth.

Also, melt in a *bain marie* a pound of sugar. Mix with the infusion and heat the preparation without bringing it to the boil. Leave to cool and then bottle. When suffering from colic take two or three tablespoonfuls of the syrup.

Juniper berry water

This is another preparation considered to be very effective in dealing with colicky pains.

Place in a receptacle with a lid 250 g of juniper berries, the zest of half a lemon, half a coffeespoonful of saffron, a pound of granulated sugar, a litre of *eau de vie* and a large glass of water. Leave to macerate for two weeks, stirring at some length once a day. Strain and press well through a fine cloth before decanting. Take a small liqueur glass of this preparation in case of colic.

Sundry methods

Potato method: make a very dry potato mash and enclose it in a piece of gauze. Apply this poultice to the abdomen.
Basil: take three cupfuls of basil infusion (preparation No. 22) in the course of the day.
Mint: when in pain, drink a cup of mint infusion (preparation No. 106).
Orange flowers: take a cup of orange flower infusion when in pain (preparation No. 119).
Verbena: take during the course of the day four cups of verbena decoction (preparation No. 164).

CHRONIC ENTERITIS

Take for ten days in the month three cups of bilberry decoction (preparation No. 112); one cup first thing in the morning, a cup in the afternoon and another one before retiring. *(Translator's note:* any diarrhoeal condition of more than forty-eight hours' duration should be reported to a doctor.)

CONSTIPATION

Constipation, due in the past to bad nutrition, was a chronic affliction and that is the reason why popular medicine, throughout the centuries, worked out many procedures for its treatment, a number of which are helpful. However, if one of these has produced a satisfactory result it should not be followed for too long and, in the event of a recurrence of constipation, another method of treatment should be tried.

Stewed pumpkin

Cut into small pieces 200 g of apples and 800 g of pumpkin. Cook on a slow fire with 100 g of sugar and just enough water to cover the fruit. When well cooked put through a sieve. Eat in lieu of breakfast.

Herb broth

Cook in a litre of water a generous handful of chervil and the same amounts of sorrel, lettuce and white beet. When cooked, add a little salt. Drink the broth first thing in the morning.

White bryony syrup

Obtain a large fresh root of white bryony. Bore with the end of a pointed knife a hole in the root several centimetres deep. Fill the hole with granulated sugar. Place the bryony in a receptacle and leave to macerate for twelve hours in a dark and damp place. Drink two tablespoonfuls of this syrup before retiring at night.

Bryony can also be used in the following way: put in a saucepan a heaped tablespoonful of dried bryony root to a litre of cold water. Cover and leave to macerate for two hours. Bring slowly to the boil several times and then remove from the heat. Leave to infuse for a quarter of an hour and strain. Take first thing in the morning a cupful of this preparation. Repeat the treatment for several consecutive days.

Stewed figs

Cook four fresh figs, cut into quarters, and a dozen dried raisins to a third of a litre of milk. Eat the stewed fruit in its juice for breakfast.

Marsh mallow enema

Mix the yolk of an egg with a coffeecup of castor oil. Incorporate with this preparation a quarter of a litre of marsh mallow root decoction (preparation No. 88). The decoction should be cool enough to avoid the risk of the egg yolk congealing. This preparation is given as an enema first thing in the morning. The temperature of the liquid should never exceed 37° C, i.e. the temperature of the body.

Stewed prunes

Soak for a day ten dried prunes in half a litre of water. Cook slowly without sugar. Simmer for ten minutes and add the juice of a lemon. Eat five stewed prunes and drink the juice half an hour before breakfast. Also drink four glasses of water between meals: two glasses in the morning and two in the afternoon. Eat two apples before retiring. Repeat the next day and if there is no improvement in the condition switch to another method on the third day.

Sundry methods

Footbath: take a footbath of tepid water before retiring. After three minutes remove part of the warm water and replace it with cold water. Wait another three minutes before repeating the procedure and so on until the feet have soaked in the bath for ten minutes.

Cornflower: take a tablespoonful of honey mixed with half a coffeespoonful of cornflower seeds first thing in the morning.

Alder buckthorn: put in a saucepan a coffeespoonful of alder buckthorn bark and a tablespoonful of dried orange zest in a litre of cold water. Bring slowly to the boil and simmer until the liquid is reduced by half. Remove the saucepan from the fire and add half a coffeespoonful of cumin seeds and leave to infuse for two hours. Strain. Drink a cup of this decoction before retiring.

Carrots: cook slowly a kilo of sliced carrots to a litre of water. When cooked, add a little salt, sieve, and eat the preparation for breakfast.

Olive oil: soak with olive oil a piece of toast and eat it at breakfast for three consecutive days.

Lettuce: drink before retiring a decoction of lettuce leaves (preparation No. 93).

Orange: boil the fresh peel of an orange for half an hour. Remove the water and cook in some fresh water with four lumps of sugar for another half an hour. Remove the orange peel and place it on a strainer to drain. Eat half before retiring and at least two hours after the evening meal, and the other half on an empty stomach in the morning.
Peach blossom: eat first thing in the morning a slice of bread spread with either butter or jam and then covered with peach blossom. Do not use this method for more than three consecutive days.
Pumpkin: drink first thing in the morning a large glass of pumpkin juice.
Liquorice: drink first thing in the morning and again before retiring at night a cup of liquorice decoction (preparation No. 134). Some might find the liquorice maceration (preparation No. 136) more helpful.
Rhubarb: take first thing in the morning a cup of rhubarb root infusion (preparation No. 139).

INTESTINAL DISORDERS

Bilberries

Take six cups of bilberry decoction (preparation No. 113) during the day. This method is particularly good in cases of intestinal infection and fermentation.

Cumin seeds

Place in a saucepan a coffeespoonful of cumin seeds. Pour on a cup of hot water. Bring slowly to the boil, leave to infuse for ten minutes and then strain.

Drink a cup of this decoction after each of the three main meals.

Coriander seeds

Place in a saucepan a coffeespoonful of coriander seeds to a cup of cold water. Bring slowly to the boil several times and then remove from the heat and leave to infuse for ten minutes before straining.

Take one cup of this preparation after each of the three main meals.

DIARRHOEA

Popular medicine has many treatments for diarrhoea but the condition itself is only a sympton. It can result from mild poisoning but can also be the sign of a more serious illness. For this reason it should always be treated with caution. If in doubt consult a doctor.

Cabbage cure

According to popular medicine cabbage is the natural remedy for those intestinal infections that give diarrhoea. Apparently a swift cure can be obtained by eating nothing but boiled cabbage, cauliflower, or uncooked sauerkraut.

Bilberry cure

Bilberry is also considered in popular medicine as a specific for those conditions that give diarrhoea.

Eat first thing in the morning a coffeecupful of fresh bilberries. At the same time take every half an hour a tablespoonful of dried bilberry decoction (preparation No. 113).

Bilberry *eau de vie* is also considered very effective. It is prepared in the following manner: drop into a litre bottle 250 g of fresh berries; fill with *eau de vie,* cork and leave to macerate in a warm place for twenty days, shaking the bottle twice a day. On the twenty-first day squeeze the berries well and strain through a fine cloth. Take a tablespoonful of this preparation immediately after breakfast, another one in the afternoon and a third before retiring.

Sundry methods

Arnica: put in a receptacle a tablespoonful of dried arnica flowers. Pour on half a litre of boiling water, stir well, cover and leave to infuse for a quarter of an hour. Strain through a cloth lined with cotton wool to trap the downy hairs of the plant. Take the preparation in small mouthfuls hourly throughout the day, drinking the equivalent of a teacupful in all.

Artichoke: take throughout the day four tablespoonfuls of artichoke maceration (preparation No. 16).
Wood avens: take two coffeespoonfuls of wood avens root tincture (preparation No. 25) during the day.
Heath: drink throughout the day four cups of heath decoction (preparation No. 38): a cup first thing in the morning, a cup in the middle of the morning, one in the middle of the afternoon and the last before retiring.
Dog rose: take three aperitif glasses of dog rose hip wine (preparation No. 74): one glass in the morning, at midday and in the evening.
Strawberry: drink a cupful of strawberry decoction (preparation No. 81) first thing in the morning and another before retiring.
Onions: peel about ten onions and put the skins in a saucepan to a litre of cold water. Bring slowly to the boil, boil for ten minutes and strain. Drink half a litre of this preparation throughout the day.
Pellitory-of-the-wall: drink three cupfuls of an infusion of pellitory-of-the-wall (preparation No. 125) throughout the day. This treatment is particularly suitable for children.
Bramble: put in a receptacle a tablespoonful of bramble leaves, pour on half a litre of boiling water, stir well, cover and leave to infuse for ten minutes before straining. Drink the infusion in several draughts during the day.
Elder: put in a receptacle two tablespoonfuls of dried elder leaves. Pour on a litre of red wine, heat slowly, remove from the heat the moment it reaches boiling point, leave to infuse for an hour and strain. Take in the course of the day several aperitif glasses of this preparation.

STOMACH ACIDITY

Rhubarb

Take before each of the main means a cupful of rhubarb infusion (preparation No. 139).

DIFFICULT DIGESTION

Angelica decoction

Place in a saucepan a glassful of fresh roots of angelica, half a litre of water and half a litre of red wine. Bring slowly to the boil, remove from the heat after having brought it to the boil two or three times, strain and bottle. Drink an aperitif glass of the decoction before the midday and evening meals.

Sauerkraut

According to popular medicine those people who have a difficult digestion should take before each meal two tablespoonfuls of uncooked sauerkraut.

Camomile infusion

With meals drink only a cupful of camomile infusion prepared in the following way: put in a cup five camomile flower heads, fill with boiling water, stir well, leave to infuse for five minutes before straining. Follow this treatment for at least one month.

Lime (linden) infusion

Drink after the midday and evening meals a cupful of lime infusion prepared in the following manner: put in a cup a heaped coffeespoonful of lime flowers, fill with boiling water, stir well, cover and leave to infuse for ten minutes before straining. Sweeten slightly and add a coffeespoonful of *eau de vie*.

STOMACH CRAMPS

Angelica

When in pain take a tablespoonful of angelica wine (preparation No. 9). If the cramps are frequent take the wine for a week at the dose of one tablespoonful before the three main meals.

Liquorice

Those prone to frequent stomach cramps should drink, until the condition has improved, a cupful of liquorice decoction (preparation No. 134) after the three main meals.

Camomile
When in pain, take a cup of camomile infusion (preparation No. 44).

STOMACH ACHE

It is impossible to know exactly what stomach ache implies when it is referred to in folk medicine. Ulcers and cramps have their specific treatment: as for any other discomfort, such as heartburn, acidity, etc., the following methods would seem to be harmless and could be resorted to when the reason for the pain is not clear. However, if the pain persists a doctor must be consulted.

Grape cure
According to popular medicine a grape cure is beneficial to the stomach. Eat a kilo of grapes a day, adding the fruit to the usual diet: take one pound an hour before breakfast (or in place of breakfast), half a pound two hours before the midday and evening meals.

Juniper berries
Take, first thing in the morning and one hour before breakfast, about a dozen juniper berries.

Sundry methods

Almond milk: when in pain drink two or three mouthfuls of almond milk (preparation No. 6).
Camomile: take each morning before breakfast, for ten days, an aperitif glass of camomile wine (preparation No. 46).
Marjoram: drink a cupful of marjoram infusion (preparation No. 99) before each of the three main meals.
Balm: at the onset of pain drink a cup of hot balm infusion (preparation No. 104).
Rosemary: drink before each of the three main meals an aperitif glass of rosemary wine (preparation No. 141).
Sage: drink after midday and evening meals a cupful of sage infusion (preparation No. 145).

Marigold: drink a cupful of marigold infusion (preparation No. 150) after each of the three main meals.
Verbena: take a cupful of verbena decoction (preparation No. 164) after each of the three main meals.

STOMACH ULCERS

Popular medicine methods for the treatment of stomach ulcers are often effective providing treatment is carried out before the condition has gone too far.

Potato juice

Drink first thing in the morning and two hours after each meal a coffeecupful of raw potato juice. Follow the treatment for one month. Potato juice can be unpleasant to the taste and to make it more palatable it can be mixed with a little honey or carrot juice.

Another way of making use of the healing properties of raw potato is to eat three grated potatoes daily but, again, to make it more palatable add some honey or carrot juice to the pulp.

Honey cure

Take a tablespoonful of honey first thing in the morning and do not eat breakfast for one hour. Follow this treatment for a week.

During the second week take two tablespoonfuls of honey two hours before breakfast and continue thus during a further fortnight.If there is no improvement after these three weeks take four tablespoonfuls of honey in the morning for another fortnight and abstain from food until lunch.

Camomile

Drink a cupful of camomile infusion (preparation No. 44) first thing in the morning and one cup after each of the three main meals. Follow the treatment for two months.

St John's wort

Take between meals four times a day a lump of sugar soaked in a little St John's wort oil (preparation No. 109).

TO PREVENT INDIGESTION

Camomile wine

Half an hour before a meal which is likely to be rich drink an aperitif glass of camomile wine (preparation No. 46).

Angelica infusion

Drink a cupful of angelica infusion (preparation No. 7) one hour before a meal that is expected to be heavy or rich. Drink another cup after the meal.

Cinnamon alcohol

This is a recipe that has to be prepared in advance and made use of when a heavy meal is in the offing.

Put in a bottle three tablespoonfuls of cinnanon and pour on a quarter of a litre of *eau de vie*. Place in another bottle three tablespoonfuls of brown sugar and an eighth of a litre of rose water. Cork both bottles and leave to macerate for twenty-four hours, shaking the bottles from time to time. Then mix the contents together and decant them into a third bottle, filtering as you do so. Cork the bottle and keep for use when needed.

Five hours before the meal, take one tablespoonful of the preparation and another two hours later.

INDIGESTION

The following methods should be resorted to at the first signs of indigestion.

Garlic broth

Whether indigestion has been checked or has been relieved by vomiting it is beneficial to take the following morning a garlic broth prepared as follows: place in a saucepan six peeled garlic cloves; pour on a litre of boiling water, boil slowly for twenty minutes and strain.

Peppercorns

At the first signs of indigestion swallow intact about a dozen peppercorns, washed down with a mouthful of wine.

Coffee and lemon

At the first signs of indigestion drink a cup of coffee to which has been added the juice of a lemon.

Vichy water and lemon

Drink the juice of a lemon and immediately afterwards a glass of Vichy water. If Vichy water is not available, take a glass of water to which has been added a quarter of a coffeespoonful of bicarbonate of soda.

Sundry infusions

Cumin: drink a cup of hot cumin infusion (preparation No. 68) and another one half an hour later.
Balm: drink a hot infusion of balm (preparation No. 104) and three more cups with an interval of one hour between each.
Tansy: drink a cupful of tansy infusion (preparation No. 153) and a second one an hour later.
Lime (linden): drink a cup of lime decoction (preparation No. 158) and another one an hour later.
Veronica: drink a cupful of veronica decoction (preparation No. 161) and follow it an hour later with three cups of veronica infusion (preparation No. 162).

LIVER DISORDERS

Popular medicine does not distinguish one liver disorder from another. The following methods may be used, however, whenever there is a liver disorder and particularly for the relief of biliousness.

Cabbage salad

Popular medicine recommends to those suffering from liver disorders, particularly from cirrhosis, a cabbage salad seasoned with olive oil and lemon juice, to be eaten at every meal.

Bicarbonate of soda bath

When a bilious attack is felt to be imminent or has even begun, take a hot bath in which has been dissolved 500 g of bicarbonate of soda.

Olive oil method

It is possible to ward off an imminent bilious attack by drinking a claret glass of olive oil. This should not be taken until the last meal eaten has been digested. In some cases drinking a glass of olive oil during the actual attack can bring relief. *(Translator's note:* these remedies are not without risk as ingestion of oil could aggravate the symptoms of an accompanying gall bladder disease.)

Application of hot compresses

Smear the hand with olive oil and massage clockwise the painful areas for a few minutes. Meanwhile, have ready at hand a few thick towels and some boiling water. Fold the towels to a size slightly larger than the area to be covered. Soak one towel in boiling water, wring it out thoroughly, lay it on a dry towel and apply to the area of the patient's liver, the hot towel next to the skin and the dry one on the outside.

Keep the towels in place for five minutes before repeating the process and make four further applications of compresses at intervals of five minutes. This method of a series of applications may be used two or three times daily.

Cabbage leaf application

Apply to the painful area two or three layers of cabbage leaves (see preparation No. 55). Hold in place with a flannel wrapped round the patient's abdomen. Renew the poultice every four hours. Before the patient goes to sleep make a thicker poultice which should be kept throughout the night.

Sundry methods

Artichoke: take a claret glass of artichoke wine, on an empty stomach in the morning and another before retiring (preparation No. 17).

Another method is to take for twelve consecutive days a cupful of artichoke decoction (preparation No. 15) one hour before the midday meal and another one before the evening meal. Drink the infusion hot and sweetened.

Box leaves: those prone to bilious attacks may benefit from

drinking a decoction of box leaves (preparation No. 41) for one week in the month. Take one cupful on an empty stomach in the morning, a cupful before the midday meal and another before retiring.
Camomile: throughout the duration of a bilious attack take instead of breakfast a cup of camomile infusion prepared in the following manner: put in a cup five camomile flower heads, fill with boiling water, stir well, cover and leave to infuse for ten minutes. Strain.
Chervil: take on an empty stomach in the morning two glasses of chervil infusion, either cold or lukewarm (preparation No. 51).
Lemon: place in a receptacle three sliced lemons, pour on a large cup of boiling water, cover and leave to macerate throughout the night. Strain the following morning and drink the preparation on an empty stomach.
Broom: take before each of the three main meals a cupful of broom flower infusion for one week in the month (preparation No. 84).
Onion: take an aperitif glass of onion wine (preparation No. 116) first thing in the morning and another before retiring.
Dandelion: throughout the duration of a liver attack take a cupful of dandelion infusion (preparation No. 129) before each of the three main meals.
Rosemary: put in a saucepan two coffeespoonfuls of rosemary and a cupful of hot water. Boil gently for five minutes and then strain. Drink every day, first thing in the morning, a cupful of this infusion hot and well sweetened.
Veronica: take a cupful of veronica decoction (preparation No. 161) a quarter of an hour before the three main meals.

NAUSEA

Salt water

Nausea can be overcome by drinking small mouthfuls of salt water – half a coffeespoonful of table salt to a glass of water.

Dog rose hips
Dog rose or wild rose hips are said to have the property of checking nausea. When feeling sick drink a cupful of rose hip decoction (preparation No. 72) and follow with a second cupful half an hour later.

Water compress
Apply to the neck of the person suffering from nausea a cloth soaked in cold water.

INTESTINAL PARASITES

The methods proposed by popular medicine for the explusion of intestinal parasites are no longer of very great interest as cheap and more palatable remedies can be bought at any pharmacy. But for the record here are a few popular medicine recommendations.

Garlic method
Throughout France for a very long time garlic has been used as a specific for the destruction of oxyuris or pinworm. The most usual method consists of putting four garlic cloves that have been grated into a cup, fill with boiling water, cover and leave to macerate throughout the night. Next morning strain and take the preparation on an empty stomach. Follow the treatment for two or three weeks.

If preferred, drink first thing in the morning a glass of milk in which two garlic cloves, cut into large pieces, have been macerating all night.

An enema may also be given: the liquid needed is half a litre of water in which two garlic cloves have been boiled for a quarter of an hour. Remember that the temperature of an enema should not exceed 37° C, i.e. body heat.

In the past necklaces of garlic were hung around children's necks as a preventive measure against pinworm.

Garlic was also sometimes used to drive out tapeworm. The method employed was as follows: boil in half a litre of milk for twenty minutes the previously grated cloves of a head of garlic. Drink the preparation every morning on an empty stomach. No food should be taken until the midday meal. Continue this treatment until satisfied that the tapeworm has been expelled.

Pumpkin seeds

Take 100 g of pumpkin or gourd seeds; remove the husks and crush the seeds together with a little granulated sugar. Take this preparation first thing in the morning and an aperient one hour later. It is said that this method is nearly always successful.

FOOD POISONING

(*Translator's note:* in the U.K. cases of bacterial food poisoning are notifiable diseases. Popular medicine suggests inducing vomiting by the patient but this is quite likely to make the condition worse. It is suggested, therefore, that the following be considered as of merely historical interest.)

The first thing to do in a case of food poisoning is to call a doctor but while waiting for qualified assistance it might help if vomiting is induced.

After vomiting it is recommended by folk medicine that a glass of olive oil or a lot of milk be drunk. We believe that it is better to do nothing except in the case where a doctor is unlikely to arrive for a long time.

White of egg method

To provoke vomiting the patient is given a large glass of tepid water in which the whites of two eggs have been beaten. The water should not be too cool but on the other hand not hot enough for the white of egg to set.

Butter method

Melt 50 g of butter and stir into a small coffeecupful of tepid water and four spoonfuls of olive oil. This mixture is given to the patient to induce vomiting.

Mustard seeds

To induce instant vomiting take half a glass of tepid water in which a coffeespoonful of ground mustard seeds has been mixed. *(Translator's note:* mustard powder, far more common in this country than in France, will do just as well BUT see note at beginning of this section on the inadvisability of inducing vomiting.)

DRUG ADDICTION

According to very ancient beliefs in folk medicine certain addictions could be broken by taking a cupful of barberry bark decoction (preparation No. 76) after each meal. This treatment, obviously, must be followed for a long time, i.e. long enough to be sure that the patient is free from addiction.

ALCOHOLIC INTOXICATION

The following is a sobering-up syrup: extract the juice from a cabbage, preferably a red one. Cook the juice with twice its weight in sugar until a fairly thick syrup is obtained. As soon as the intoxicating effect of alcohol is felt take two tablespoonfuls of the syrup followed by a third half an hour later.

ALCOHOLISM

The following preparation is said to possess the property of checking the urge to drink.

Put in a saucepan five tablespoonfuls of parsley leaves, the rind of a grapefruit and the zest of an orange, both of which have been cut into small pieces, and a litre of cold water. Bring slowly to the boil and leave to boil until the volume of the liquid has been reduced by half. Press well and strain through a cloth. A coffeespoonful of this preparation should be taken first thing each morning.

SCURVY

The methods proposed by popular medicine to treat scurvy have lost much of their importance since cheap and effective remedies with a vitamin C basis may be bought in any pharmacy. Furthermore, fresh fruit is available now all the year round in most places. It is interesting, however, to examine the methods popular medicine recorded.

An aperitif glass of watercress wine (preparation No. 67) to be taken before each of the three main meals is supposed to be particularly effective in fighting scurvy. Also recommended is dog rose hip syrup liqueur (preparation No. 73) of which the dose is one liqueur glass to be taken after each of the three main meals.

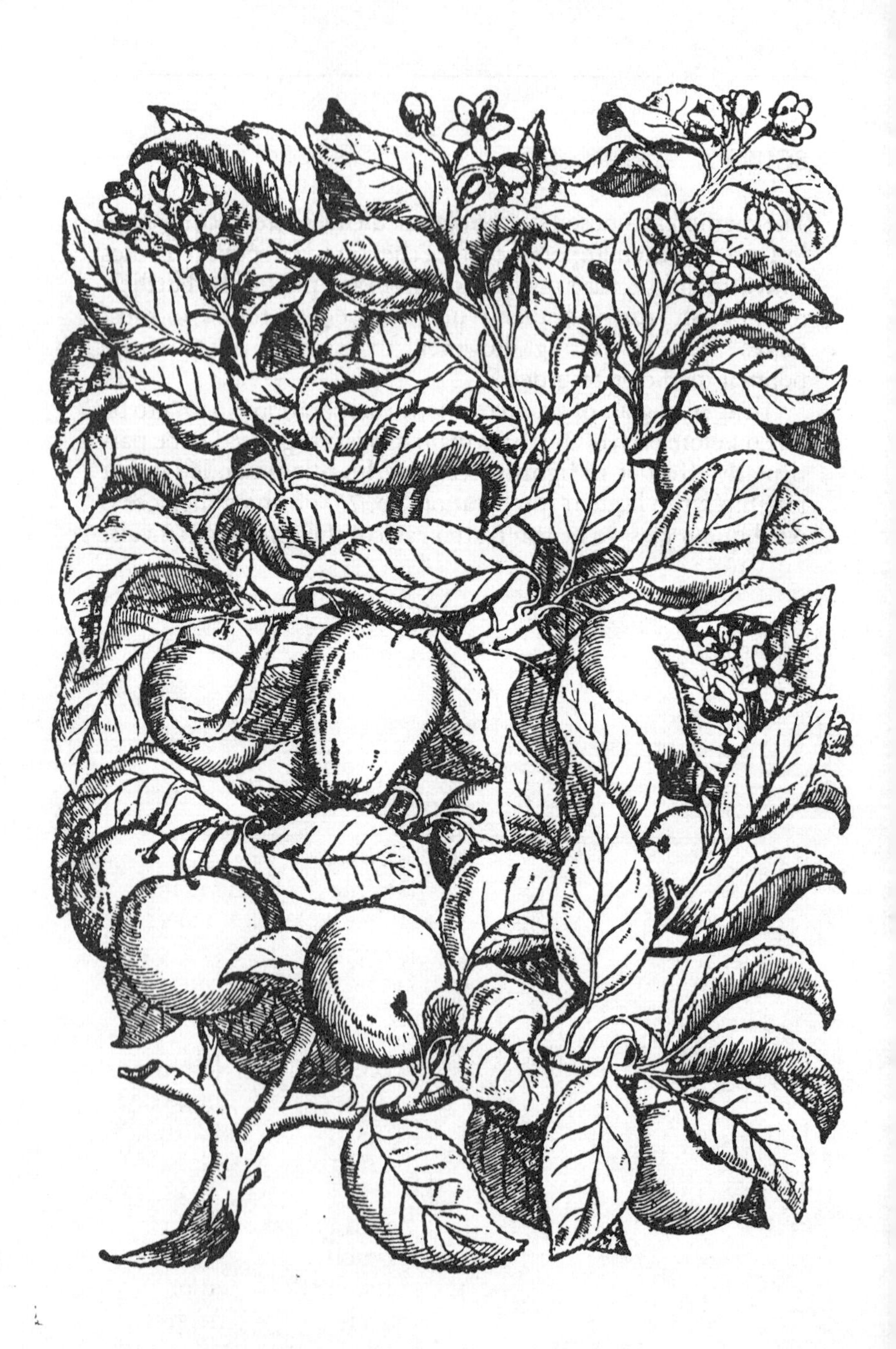

The Urinary Tract

Under this heading will be found not only those disorders that affect the urinary tract but also those that reveal their presence by changes in the urine itself.

PROTEINURIA · CALCULIA · RENAL COLIC
CYSTITIS · DIABETES · PROSTATIC PAIN
LOIN PAINS · URAEMIA · BLADDER DISORDERS
INFLAMMATION OF THE URINARY TRACT
INCONTINENCE OF URINE · RETENTION OF URINE
BLOOD IN THE URINE

PROTEINURIA

Bean pod infusion

Popular medicine has always set much store by bean pods for lowering the albumin level.

Take an infusion of bean pods (preparation No. 91) twice a day: one cupful between breakfast and the midday meal and the other between the midday and evening meals.

The infusion can also be prepared in the following manner: place in a large cup four French or runner bean pods that have been cut into small pieces; fill with boiling water, stir well, cover and leave to infuse for ten minutes before straining.

Sundry methods

Blackcurrant: drink an infusion of blackcurrant leaves four times a day (preparation No. 49): a cupful one hour before breakfast, another between breakfast and lunch, a third between lunch and the evening meal, and a fourth on retiring and at least two hours after supper.
Broom: take during one week in the month an infusion of broom (preparation No. 84): one cupful after each of the main meals.
Bittersweet: take a decoction of bittersweet (preparation No. 69): one cupful after the three main meals.

CALCULIA (STONES)

The following folk medicine remedies have the reputation of dispersing stones in whatever part of the urinary tract they may be situated. The methods may therefore be used in all cases of lithiasis.

Bean meal

Dry thoroughly in the oven some broad bean pods and grind them to a fine powder in a mixer. Take each morning a quarter of a coffeespoonful of this powder in a little wine.

Olive oil

Take first thing in the morning a tablespoonful of olive oil mixed with the juice of half a lemon.

Watercress juice and hazel nuts

Drink first thing in the morning a glass of watercress juice (most easily obtained by putting the cress through a mixer). Also eat 100 g of hazel nuts each day between meals.

Onion and alder buckthorn

Brown a large sliced onion in four tablespoonfuls of olive oil. When the onions are fried to a golden brown pour into the saucepan a glass of water and add a large spoonful of lard. Boil this mixture for ten minutes and strain.

Drink this liquid very hot and unsalted before the evening meal. Two hours later take a cupful of alder buckthorn decoction (preparation No. 34).

Sundry methods

Cherry stalks: take a decoction of cherry stalks four times a day: a cupful first thing in the morning, a cupful in the course of the morning, one in the afternoon and a fourth before retiring (preparation No. 52).

Horsetail: put in a saucepan four tablespoonfuls of dried horsetail stalks to half a litre of water. Bring slowly to the boil, boil for half an hour and strain. Drink the whole of this preparation during the day, taking it in three separate draughts.

Also prepare, for use first thing in the morning, a decoction of horsetail with two litres of water (preparation No. 130). Pour this while very hot into a bidet or similar appropriate vessel and expose the lower part of the body to the steam.
Dandelion: take a cupful of dandelion decoction after each of the three main meals (preparation No. 128).

RENAL COLIC

Olive oil enema

An olive oil enema is considered by popular medicine to be most effective in easing the pain caused by renal colic.

According to the weight of the patient the quantity of olive oil needed is between 300 g and 500 g; the oil is warmed in a *bain marie* to a temperature of 37° C before use. *(Translator's note:* this method can be very harmful to the gut and is better not attempted.)

Sundry methods

Apples: cut into slices an unpeeled apple and put the slices into a receptacle into which is then poured half a litre of boiling water. Stir, cover and leave to infuse for two hours. Press and strain the apples through a cloth. Drink the infusion at will, very hot and sweetened to taste.
Cherry stalks: take four cupfuls each day of a decoction of cherry stalks (preparation No. 52).
Cabbage: apply several layers of cabbage leaves to the painful area (see preparation No. 55).
Garlic: slice finely four cloves of garlic: put them in a receptacle with a litre of boiling water, stir well and leave to infuse for a quarter of an hour before straining. Drink this infusion whenever in pain.

CYSTITIS

Leek broth and poultice

According to popular medicine, leeks are particularly effective in the treatment of cystitis.

Take during the course of the cystitis attack three cupfuls per day of a highly concentrated leek broth made in the proportion of a pound of leeks to a litre of unsalted water. Also cook slowly a pound of leeks in olive oil. When thoroughly cooked the leeks should be mashed and wrapped in a piece of gauze of an appropriate size for application as a poultice to the lower abdomen. Keep the poultice there until it is cold.

Heath

Heath is also considered by popular medicine to be a specific for cystitis.

Take one hour before breakfast a tablespoonful of heather honey.

In addition prepare a heath infusion in the following manner: place in a receptacle three tablespoonfuls of flowering sprigs of heath; pour on a litre of boiling water, stir well and leave to infuse for ten minutes. Strain. Drink a litre of this infusion in the course of the day.

Lastly, douche twice a day with a heath decoction (preparation No. 38), taking care that the liquid is no hotter than 37°C.

Sundry methods

Camomile: prepare three litres of an infusion of camomile (preparation No. 45). Pour while hot into a receptacle and expose the lower part of the abdomen to the steam.
Blackcurrant: take four cupfuls of a decoction of blackcurrant leaves each day (preparation No. 49): one cupful first thing in the morning, a second between breakfast and luncheon, a third in the middle of the afternoon and the last before retiring.
Liquorice: take several small cupfuls a day of liquorice decoction (preparation No. 134) between meals.
Violets: take five cupfuls of violet decoction (preparation No. 167) each day between meals.

DIABETES

Bilberries are considered by popular medicine to be the specific for diabetes. Diabetics are advised to eat daily some uncooked bilberries or some bilberry jam and also to drink a litre of an infusion with a bilberry leaf basis (preparation No. 112).

The following infusion can also be prepared: place in a receptacle a tablespoonful of bilberry leaves and a tablespoonful of strawberry leaves; pour on a litre of boiling water, stir well, cover and leave to infuse ten minutes before straining. Drink all of the liquid obtained, slightly sweetened with honey, during the course of the day.

Another infusion, said to be very effective, is made in the following way: place in a saucepan a tablespoonful of bilberry leaves, a tablespoonful of eucalyptus leaves, three-quarters of a tablespoonful of valerian root and a litre of water. Bring slowly to the boil, boil for five minutes and strain. Take a cupful of this decoction first thing in the morning, another one a quarter of an hour before the midday meal and a third cupful before the evening meal.

Olive leaf infusion

Place in a saucepan two tablespoonfuls of olive leaves that have been cut into small pieces. Add a litre of cold water, cover and leave to macerate throughout the night. Next morning heat the preparation slowly and remove from the heat when it reaches boiling point. Leave to infuse for twenty minutes and then strain.

Drink the infusion in four separate draughts during the day: first thing in the morning, between the main meals and before retiring.

Sundry methods

Potatoes: drink four coffeecupfuls of potato juice each day: one first thing in the morning, a second during the course of the morning, a third during the afternoon and the last one on retiring. The juice must always be fresh and prepared immediately before it is needed. The most convenient way of doing this is by using a mixer. To disguise the unpleasantly flat taste of potato juice some lemon juice can be added to it.

Nettles: take a quarter of an hour before each of the three main meals a cupful of stinging nettle decoction (preparation No. 123).

Bean pods: drink four cupfuls daily of a French or runner bean pod decoction (preparation No. 91): one cupful first thing in the morning, one during the course of the morning, one between the two main meals and the last one before retiring.
Walnut leaves: take a cupful of walnut leaf infusion (preparation No. 115) first thing in the morning and last thing at night.

PROSTATIC PAIN

Heath infusion

Put in a saucepan eight tablespoonfuls of dried heath flowers to a litre of cold water. Bring slowly to the boil and keep it on the boil until the liquid has been reduced to half its original volume and then strain. Drink the preparation in three separate draughts during the day.

Cabbage poultice

Apply cabbage leaves to the painful areas (preparation No. 55) and hold them in place with a crêpe bandage or flannel. If the pain persists renew the poultice every two hours.

LOIN PAINS

Borage compresses

Put in a saucepan ten tablespoonfuls of dried borage to a litre of cold water. Bring slowly to the boil, boil for ten minutes and strain. When the liquid has cooled a little, soak compresses in it and apply to the painful area. Cover with a warm flannel and maintain for a good hour. Apply the compresses several times daily.

Sundry methods

Heath: take four cupfuls of heath decoction (preparation No. 38) during the day: one on an empty stomach, one during the morning, one in the afternoon and the last before retiring.
Strawberry: take a litre of strawberry root decoction (preparation No. 81) during the day: one cupful first thing in the morning,

the rest between meals during the day.
Broom: one hour before each of the main meals take a cupful of broom flower infusion (preparation No. 84). Follow the treatment for one week and repeat after an interval of a fortnight.
Onion wine: drink an aperitif glass of onion wine (preparation No. 116) first thing in the morning.
Parsley: drink one hour after each of the main meals a cupful of parsley infusion (preparation No. 126).

URAEMIA

According to folk medicine those people prone to uraemia could alleviate the condition considerably by taking a large cupful of herb broth (preparation No. 92) with each of the two main meals. Add to the broth two tablespoonfuls of finely chopped raw onion.

BLADDER DISORDERS

Black radish juice

To a glass of black radish juice add a tablespoonful of honey, stirring until it is thoroughly dissolved. Take for four days first thing in the morning a glass of this preparation.

INFLAMMATION OF THE URINARY TRACT

St John's wort

Drink half a coffeecupful of St John's wort and stinging nettle infusion (preparation No. 110) every two hours but abstain during the hour before a meal and for two hours after a meal.

Horsetail decoction

Take an hour after each of the three main meals a cupful of horsetail decoction (preparation No. 130).

INCONTINENCE OF URINE

The belt method

According to folk medicine incontinence is encouraged by sleeping on the back and it is therefore suggested that at night a belt be worn which has something hard, e.g. a cork, fixed at the back. If the patient turns on to his back while asleep the discomfort of the cork pressing into his back will cause him to turn automatically on to his side.

Horsetail decoction

Take two hours before retiring a cupful of horsetail decoction (preparation No. 130).

Bilberry decoction

Place in a saucepan three tablespoonfuls of bilberry leaves to a litre of cold water. Bring to the boil and leave to boil slowly until the liquid is reduced by one third. Strain and give the patient two coffeecupfuls of the decoction, well sweetened, before he retires.

RETENTION OF URINE

Leek poultice

Cook over mild heat (according to popular medicine an earthenware vessel should be used) six leeks just covered with olive oil. When the leeks are well cooked wrap them in gauze and apply to the lower abdomen. Leave the poultice in place until it is cold.

Watercress juice

Extract the juice from some watercress and mix with it an equal quantity of olive oil. Drink a glass of this preparation when in pain.

Onion juice

It is easier to extract the juice of onions if they have been chopped first. To half a glass of onion juice add a similar amount of white wine. Mix thoroughly and drink a glass of the preparation first thing in the morning.

Nettle juice

Extract half a glass of juice from some fresh stinging nettles. Mix with the juice an equal amount of white wine. Drink a glass of this preparation on an empty stomach every morning.

Sundry methods

Peaches: take a glass of peach juice first thing every morning for a week.

Birch infusion: take three cupfuls of birch infusion (preparation No. 32) each day: a cupful in the middle of the morning, one in the middle of the afternoon and the third before retiring. This treatment should be followed for at least one month.

Heath: drink each day a litre and a half of a decoction of heath, strawberry-tree leaves and white deadnettles (preparation No. 40): one cupful first thing in the morning and the remainder in draughts spaced well away from meals throughout the day. Follow the treatment for a fortnight with a lapse of a fortnight before repeating it and so on in alternating fortnights.

Wild carrots: take a cupful of wild carrot decoction before each of the three main meals (preparation No. 47).

Blackcurrant: take four cupfuls of blackcurrant leaf decoction each day (preparation No. 49): a cupful first thing in the morning, one the middle of the morning, one in the middle of the afternoon and the last one before retiring.

Cherry stalks: take four cupfuls each day of cherry stalk decoction (preparation No. 52) between meals.

Rose hip: take a litre of wild rose hip decoction (preparation No. 72) in the form of several draughts throughout the day.

French beans: take first thing in the morning a glass of the juice of French or dwarf beans.

Parsley: take four cupfuls of parsley infusion (preparation No. 126) each day: a cupful on an empty stomach, one mid-morning, one mid-afternoon and the fourth one hour before bedtime.

Violets: take four cupfuls of violet decoction (preparation No. 167) each day: one first thing in the morning, one two hours before the midday meal, one two hours before the evening meal and the fourth before retiring.

BLOOD IN THE URINE

Powdered vine leaves

Dry some vine leaves in the oven and crush them with a rolling pin or bottle. Drink a large cupful of vegetable broth to which a small coffeespoonful of this powder has been added. *(Translator's note:* haematuria (bloodstained urine) is a grave clinical sign which should be reported immediately to a doctor.)

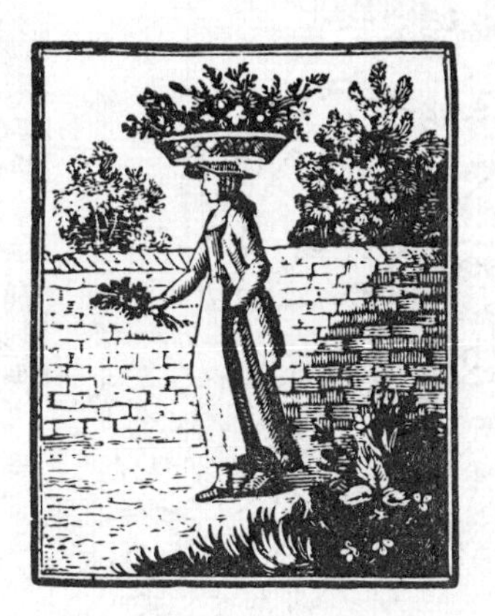

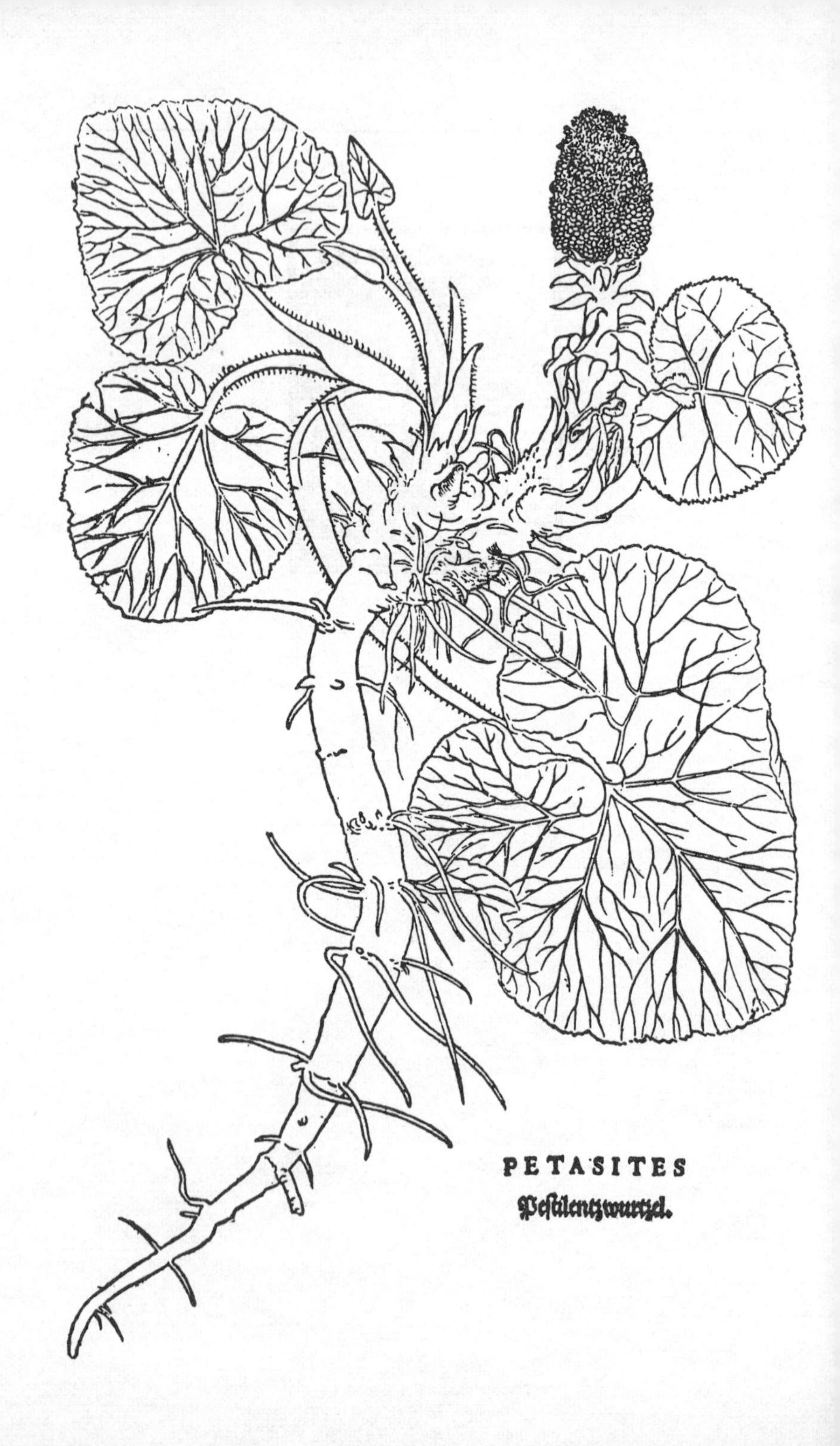
PETASITES
Pestilentzwurtzel.

Childhood Diseases

WHOOPING COUGH · MEASLES
SCARLET FEVER · CHICKEN POX

WHOOPING COUGH

Turnip syrup

Wash and dry some unpeeled turnips and cut them in slices. Place them in a colander suspended over a bowl; sprinkle the turnips with plenty of sugar and leave to macerate for a few hours. Collect the juice from the bowl and give it to the child in doses of one coffeespoonful every hour.

Garlic maceration

Chop finely three garlic heads. Put the garlic in a receptacle and pour on a quarter of a litre of boiling water. Cover and leave to macerate for a whole day. Filter the preparation. Give the child one tablespoonful of this preparation every two hours.

Leek syrup

Cut into thick slices the white part of three large leeks. Boil slowly for twenty minutes in half a litre of water. Press well and strain the leeks through a cloth and add to the liquid nine lumps of sugar. Give the preparation to the patient in small cupfuls throughout the day.

Carrot syrup

Use a mixer, if possible, to extract the juice from a pound of carrots. Boil slowly until the liquid is reduced by half. Add several lumps of sugar and give the child a coffeespoonful of the syrup every hour.

Hazel nut infusion

Place in a litre of boiling water a score of hazel nuts that have been shelled but not cut or crushed. Allow to simmer gently until the liquid is reduced to about a third of a litre. Strain and give the infusion hot to the patient.

Sundry methods

Basil: place in a receptacle three tablespoonfuls of basil. Pour on a litre of boiling water. Stir well, cover and leave to infuse for five minutes. Strain. The infusion should be drunk at frequent intervals throughout the day, particularly at the onset of coughing.
Poppy: Three cupfuls of poppy infusion (preparation No. 65) to be taken each day: one first thing in the morning, one before lunch and the third before retiring.
Fennel: take a cupful of fennel infusion (preparation No. 80) before each of the three main meals.
Lavender: drink an infusion of lavender flowers (preparation No. 94a), four cupfuls a day between meals.
Rosemary: when there is a fit of coughing drink a small cupful of rosemary infusion (preparation No. 140).

The following infusion is said to have a very beneficial action: place in a receptacle a tablespoonful of rosemary, a tablespoonful of basil and two tablespoonfuls of thyme; pour on a litre of boiling water; stir well, cover and leave to infuse for ten minutes. Strain and add two tablespoonfuls of honey; take half a coffeecupful of this preparation every half hour.
Violets: take five cupfuls daily of violet decoction (preparation No. 167) between meals.

MEASLES

Although measles is generally a mild illness, a doctor should always be called. Just the same it can be helpful to get the patient to drink an elder flower infusion (preparation No. 152) or a borage infusion with a coffeespoonful of honey stirred into each cup. Some traditions recommend that milk be added to borage infusion in measles cases.

SCARLET FEVER

If scarlet fever is not properly treated serious complications may arise and it is preferable not to rely on popular medicine alone for treatment. However, in addition to the medication prescribed by the doctor one can give the patient a borage infusion (preparation No. 36) in which a coffeespoonful of honey has been dissolved or milk can be added if preferred. This preparation may be drunk as frequently as wished and is said to assist recovery from scarlet fever.

CHICKEN POX

Even though chicken pox is not a serious illness a doctor should be called but to the treatment prescribed the following infusion can be given and is said to be helpful. Place in a receptacle two tablespoonfuls of dried marigold leaves or flowers. Pour on a litre of boiling water, stir well, cover and leave to infuse ten minutes before straining. The patient may drink this infusion freely.

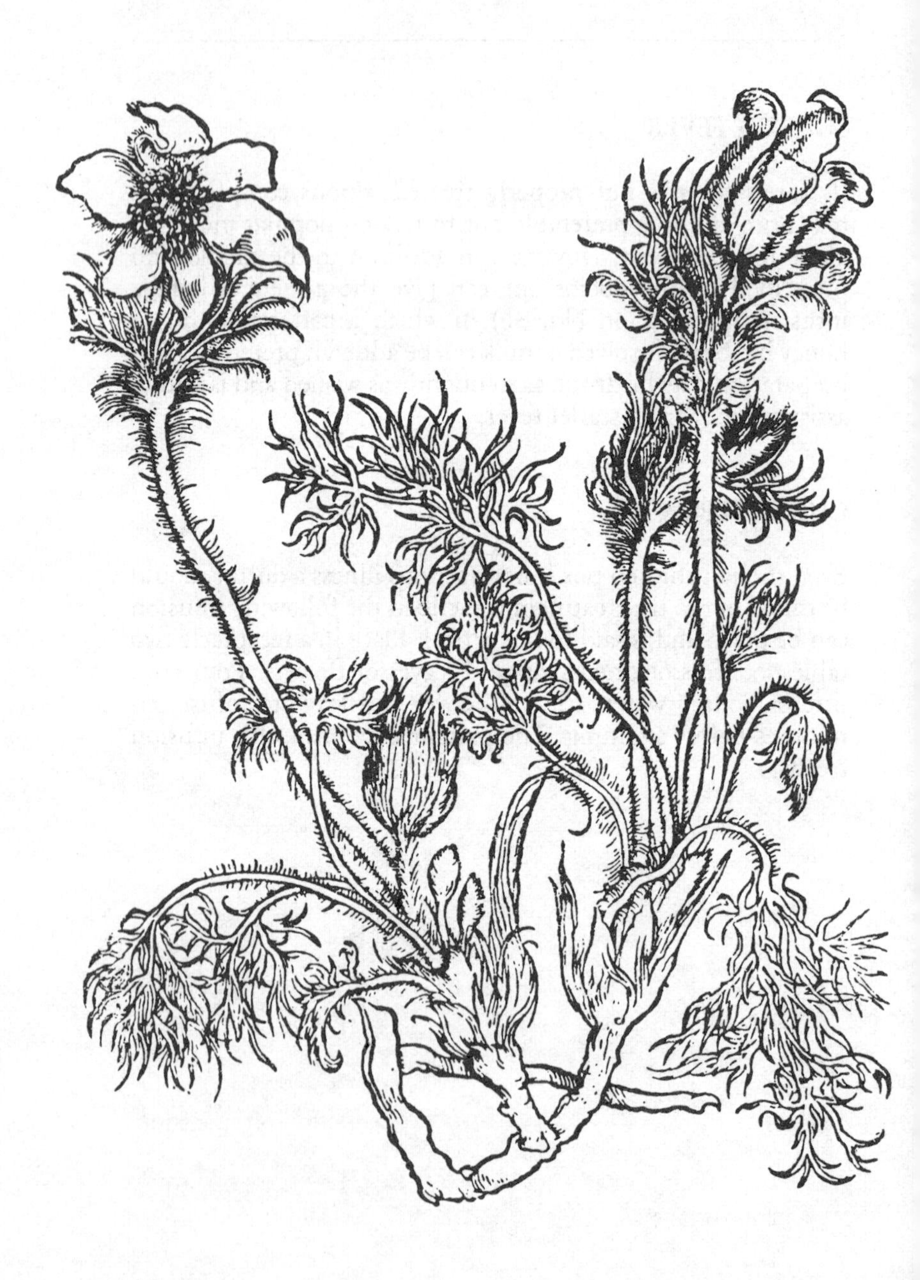

Women's Ailments

LEUCORRHOEA · METRITIS · SALPINGITIS
FIBROIDS · PAINFUL BREAST · DELAYED PERIODS
PAINFUL PERIODS · EXCESSIVELY HEAVY PERIODS
TOO FREQUENT PERIODS · IRREGULAR PERIODS
EXCESSIVELY LIGHT PERIODS
INTERRUPTION OF PERIODS · STERILITY
POST-MISCARRIAGE COMPLICATIONS
PREPARATION FOR LABOUR · TO STOP LACTATION
TO INCREASE LACTATION · PREGNANCY MARKS
MENOPAUSAL DISORDERS

LEUCORRHOEA

Popular medicine treats leucorrhoea ('whites') mainly with douches. The temperature of the douche liquid should not exceed 37° C.

Oak

Oak bark is considered the specific for leucorrhoea by popular medicine.

Douche with a decoction of oak bark morning and evening (preparation No. 58). Also drink before each of the three main meals some oak leaf decoction (preparation No. 57).

Sundry methods

Lady's smock: take a cupful of infusion of lady's smock (preparation No. 3) before the two main meals. Follow the treatment for a month.

Heath: take a cupful of heath decoction (preparation No. 38) before each of the three main meals.

Bittersweet: take a cupful of bittersweet decoction (preparation No. 69) before the three main meals.

Lavender: douche twice a day with a lavender decoction prepared in the following manner: place in a saucepan a coffee-cupful of lavender flowers to half a litre of cold water; bring slowly to the boil, boil for ten minutes, strain and add half a litre of boiling water.

Elm: douche morning and night with an elm decoction (preparation No. 121).
White deadnettle: drink morning and night a white deadnettle decoction (preparation No. 124). This plant must not be confused with the stinging nettle.
Stinging nettle: put in a bottle a coffeecupful of stinging nettle flowers; add a glass of *eau de vie* and top up the bottle with white wine. Leave to macerate for a week, shaking the bottle twice a day, and then strain. Drink first thing in the morning an aperitif glass of this preparation.
Sage: douche with sage infusion morning and night (preparation No. 145).
Tansy: drink a cup of tansy infusion before each of the three main meals (preparation No. 153).

METRITIS

The classical remedy in popular medicine for the treatment of metritis is a white deadnettle douche given morning and night. The liquid should not be hotter than 37° C.

SALPINGITIS

Prepare the following infusion: place in a receptacle a coffeespoonful of valerian root, a coffeespoonful of balm and a coffeespoonful of flowering sprigs of basil; pour on half a litre of boiling water, stir well, cover and leave to infuse for ten minutes before straining.

When in pain take the infusion but never more than three cupfuls in one day.

FIBROIDS

Lady's smock douche

Prepare a decoction in the following way: toss into a saucepan three tablespoonfuls of flowering tips of lady's smock with a litre of boiling water, stir with a spoon, boil for a quarter of an hour and strain.

Do not use until the liquid has cooled to body temperature, i.e. 37° C. Douche with this preparation three times a week.

PAINFUL BREAST

The popular medicine procedures described hereafter can be used for any painful breast condition, e.g. inflammation, congestion or cracked skin but only if the pain is occasional. Should it become chronic a doctor should be consulted.

Basil water

Put in a litre bottle five tablespoonfuls of basil; fill the bottle with rose water; leave to macerate for forty-eight hours, shaking the bottle from time to time, then strain.

Apply to the breast compresses soaked in this preparation.

Chervil poultice

Cut finely with scissors a handful of chervil. Heat it dry and by itself in a frying-pan and wrap it in a piece of gauze. Apply to the breast as a poultice and cover with a towel.

Honey poultice

Beat in an earthenware vessel the yolks of six eggs with half a pound of honey and add, little by little, three-quarters of a litre of white wine until a smooth paste is obtained. Bring slowly to the boil, stirring continually, and boil until nearly all the wine has evaporated and the preparation has the consistency of an ointment. When it has cooled, wrap the ointment in a gauze and apply the compress to the breast.

Mullein

Boil slowly for ten minutes in milk some fresh mullein leaves. Cool the preparation and apply to the breast. This treatment has the reputation of being most effective in cases of cracked skin and chapping on the breast.

Raw carrots

Apply to the breast a poultice of grated raw carrots: after about twenty minutes rinse with cold water to which has been added a dash of 90° alcohol.

Raspberry leaves

Toss into boiling milk some fresh raspberry leaves and let them simmer for five minutes. Apply them, wrapped in a towel, to the breast and keep the poultice in place for about twenty minutes.

Blackcurrant leaf infusion

When the breasts are congested take a cup of blackcurrant leaf infusion (preparation No. 49) after each of the three main meals.

DELAYED PERIODS

To bring on menstruation drink three cupfuls of mugwort infusion between meals (preparation No. 13).

In some regions of France mugwort is credited with abortifacient properties. This belief is unfounded because, on the contrary, in popular medicine mugwort was administered to women prone to miscarriages.

PAINFUL PERIODS

Mugwort decoction

A mugwort and shepherd's purse decoction (preparation No. 14) has the reputation of acting as an analgesic in cases of painful menstruation. As soon as pain is felt take a large hot cupful of the preparation and another one an hour later. Follow the treatment for three more days, taking a cupful in the morning and another an hour later.

Wood avens

When in pain drink a coffeecupful of wood avens (preparation No. 24). No more than four cups should be taken in any one day.

If the pain lessens drink in subsequent days one cup in the morning and one in the afternoon.

Mullein

Boil some mullein leaves in milk for fifteen minutes. Wrap them in a gauze and apply as a poultice to the lower abdomen.

Camomile

Whenever in pain drink a cup of hot camomile infusion (preparation No. 44).

Parsley

Extract the juice from a bunch of fresh parsley.

Also prepare the following infusion: place in a receptacle a small tablespoonful of lime (linden) flowers, a small tablespoonful of camomile flowers and the same amounts of orange flowers and balm flowers and leaves. Pour on a litre of boiling water, stir well, cover and leave to infuse for five minutes before straining.

At the first indication of pain take a coffeespoonful of parsley juice and one hour later drink the hot infusion; wait a further hour before taking another coffeespoonful of parsley and repeat the treatment every hour.

Rosemary wine

Take an aperitif glass of rosemary wine (preparation No. 141) before each of the three main meals.

Sage infusion

Drink sage infusion during the week preceding menstruation (preparation No. 145): one cupful before each of the three main meals.

EXCESSIVELY HEAVY PERIODS

Shepherd's purse

During menstruation take a tablespoonful of shepherd's purse wine every hour (preparation No. 36a).

The following decoction can also be prepared: place in a saucepan five tablespoonfuls of dried shepherd's purse stalks and flowers to a litre of cold water. Soak for an hour and bring slowly to the boil, cook for two minutes and infuse for a quarter of an hour. Strain.

Drink a cupful of this preparation before the main meals during the ten days preceding the onset of menstruation.

Oak bark

During menstruation take half a coffeespoonful of oak bark ground to a powder and mixed with a spoonful of honey. Also drink a cupful of oak bark decoction (preparation No. 58) in the course of the morning and another one in the afternoon. Oak bark mixed with comfrey is also given as a lukewarm douche on the day preceding the onset of the period and during the first three days of menstruation (preparation No. 60).

Nettle decoction

Take during menstruation a cupful of stinging nettle decoction (preparation No. 123) after the three main meals.

Horsetail decoction

During the ten days preceding menstruation take four cupfuls of horsetail decoction (preparation No. 130): a cup on rising, another during the morning, a further cup during the afternoon and a fourth at bedtime.

TOO FREQUENT PERIODS

To regularize too frequent periods drink for one week, beginning ten days after the onset of the last period, a cupful of strawberry leaf infusion (preparation No. 82), taking one cup after breakfast and another after dinner.

IRREGULAR PERIODS

Parsley infusion

Take a cupful of parsley infusion (preparation No. 126) before each of the two main meals, starting three days before the date at which the period should normally begin and continuing during the first two days of the period.

EXCESSIVELY LIGHT PERIODS

Chervil infusion

Take each day for one week a cupful of chervil infusion (preparation No. 51) after the three main meals, starting eighteen days after the onset of the last period.

Mint wine

Take first thing in the morning an aperitif glass of mint wine (preparation No. 107), starting ten days before the expected period and continuing daily until it begins.

INTERRUPTION OF PERIODS

To assure the resumption of a period that has been interrupted accidentally, e.g. by a cold or by emotional strain, take three cupfuls of mugwort infusion (preparation No. 13) daily, between meals.

STERILITY

According to popular medicine, when a woman wishes to be in a condition most favourable to conception she should eat, at the appropriate time of the month, an omelette into which two tablespoonfuls of chopped mugwort leaves have been beaten in with the eggs.

POST-MISCARRIAGE COMPLICATIONS

According to popular medicine, some post-miscarriage complications could be avoided by drinking daily two cupfuls of lady's mantle infusion (preparation No. 3): one cup during the morning and another in the afternoon.

PREPARATION FOR LABOUR

Popular medicine believes that the addition to the diet of cloves during the last three months of pregnancy can greatly ease labour.

Cloves can be given in soups or mixed with solid food. Take care to use only one clove in each dish because of its very strong flavour.

During the last week preceding labour drink two or three cupfuls daily of clove infusion. This is prepared by pouring a litre of boiling water on a coffeecupful of cloves.

Sage is also supposed to have properties as a pre-natal tonic. To prepare an infusion put in a receptacle two tablespoonfuls of sage leaves, pour on a litre of boiling water, stir well, cover, leave to infuse for ten minutes and strain. On the eighth month of pregnancy take a cupful of this preparation after each of the three main meals.

TO STOP LACTATION

According to popular medicine, carrot juice will stop lactation. Drink one glass of carrot juice first thing in the morning on four consecutive days.

The same properties are attributed to hart's tongue infusion which is prepared in the following way: put in a saucepan two tablespoonfuls of hart's tongue fronds, pour on a litre of boiling water, stir well, cover and allow to infuse for ten minutes. Strain. Drink four cupfuls of this infusion between meals. Follow this treatment for a week.

TO INCREASE LACTATION

According to popular medicine, fennel has the properties of increasing lactation. A fennel infusion is prepared in the following way: place in a receptacle two tablespoonfuls of fennel seeds, pour on a litre of boiling water, stir well, cover and leave to infuse for ten minutes. Strain.

Drink four cupfuls of the preparation daily, between meals.

PREGNANCY MARKS

The following preparation is said to hasten the fading of pregnancy marks.

Place in a receptacle six tablespoonfuls of parsley. Pour on a litre of boiling water, stir well, cover and leave to infuse for ten minutes. Add the juice of a lemon and strain. Use the preparation as a lotion morning and night.

MENOPAUSAL DISORDERS

Barberrry decoction

Take four cupfuls a day, for ten days in the month, of an infusion of the fruits of the barberry shrub (preparation No. 75): one cupful in the morning on an empty stomach, one between breakfast and the midday meal, another between lunch and supper and the fourth at bedtime.

Couchgrass decoction

Take for one week in the month a cupful of couchgrass decoction (preparation No. 61) after midday meal and evening meal.

Sage infusion

Take every other week, before the main meals of each day, a cupful of sage infusion (preparation No. 145).

Valerian infusion

Take three cupfuls daily of valerian infusion (preparation No. 160): one cup first thing in the morning, one before lunch and the third before the evening meal. Drink the infusion for ten consecutive days, stop for ten days and then resume for a further ten days, following this alternating method until the disorder has been suppressed.

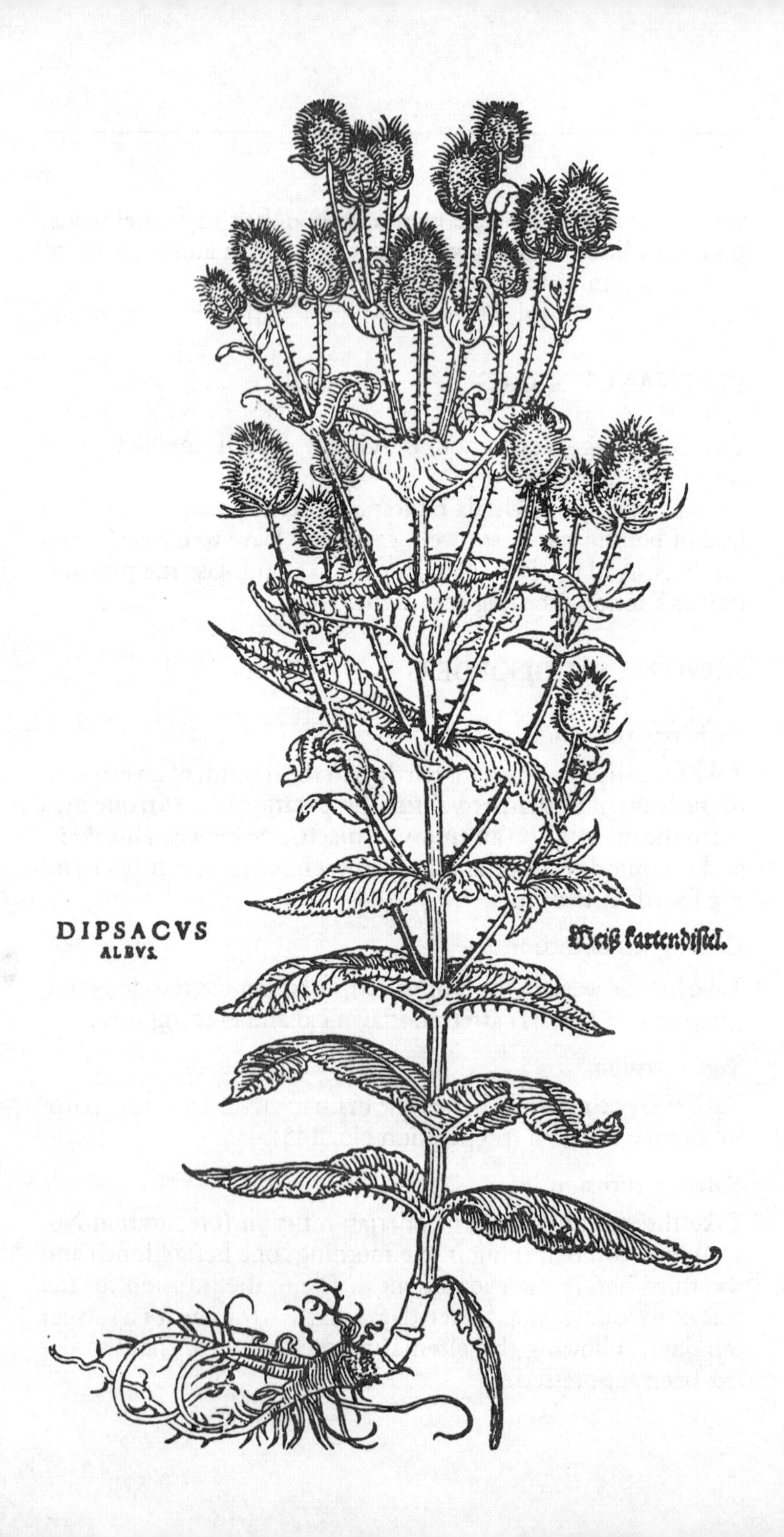
DIPSACVS
ALBVS.
Weiß kartendistel.

Sundry Disorders and Illnesses

SLIMMING METHODS · ANAEMIA · GONORRHOEA
CANCER · CELLULITE · SCROFULA · TIDEDNESS · FEVER
TYPHOID FEVER · GOITRE · DROPSY · IMPOTENCE · WENS
MENINGITIS · MALARIA · DISORDERS OF THE SPLEEN
EXCESSIVE PERSPIRATION

SLIMMING METHODS

Keeping one's figure is a comparatively modern preoccupation. In the past plumpness was often considered synonymous with beauty and consequently popular medicine offers few slimming aids but, such as they are, they are usually found to be effective.

Lemon preparations

1. Take in the morning instead of breakfast the juice of three lemons in which four coffeespoonfuls of granulated sugar have been dissolved. This method is said to bring very satisfactory results after a month.

2. Place in a mug a sliced lemon and two camomile heads. Fill with boiling water, cover and leave to macerate throughout the night. Strain off the liquid the following morning and drink it before breakfast.

3. Place in a saucepan two sliced oranges and six sliced lemons. Pour on a litre of boiling water, boil slowly for fifteen minutes and add three tablespoonfuls of honey, boil again for five minutes, stirring constantly. Strain and leave to cool. Drink a glass of this preparation first thing in the morning, another during the day and a third before retiring.

Sundry methods

Ash: take three cupfuls (one first thing in the morning, the others during the day) of a decoction of ash bark (preparation No. 83).

Grapes: when grapes are in season eat, on one day of the week, a

kilo of grapes divided into three and taken during the day in place of the normal meals.
Vine leaves: drink a cupful of vine leaf decoction (preparation No. 166) after the three main meals.

ANAEMIA

In the past mothers were frequently preoccupied by the question of anaemia in their children and therefore one finds in popular medicine many methods for dealing with it. Some of the methods act directly by fortifying the system, others act indirectly by stimulating the appetite.

Rusty wine

Put in a receptacle about ten rusty nails to a litre of white wine. Leave the vessel uncovered for three days and nights but place over the top a muslin or mesh guard against insects and dust. Strain through a fine cloth and drink a small aperitif glass of this wine first thing in the morning and last thing at night.

Cabbage salad

Take before each meal about 100 g of chopped raw cabbage, either green or red, and seasoned with the juice of a lemon.

Nettles

Mix with the food of each meal about a dozen chopped stinging nettle leaves. These can be mixed with whatever your normal food is.

Lemon cure

Take for one month the following cure, preferably in spring or autumn.

During the first week drink, half an hour before breakfast, the juice of half a lemon. During the second week drink the juice of one lemon each morning, in the third week the juice of one and a half lemons daily and in the fourth week the juice of two lemons.

Sundry methods

Wormwood: this method is considered very effective but wormwood is difficult to procure. *(Translator's note:* this is the herb – *absinthe* in French – that gave its name to the notorious aperitif beloved by French intellectuals and workers alike until it was banned by the Government in 1915 because of the ravages caused by the widespread addiction to it. That is why it has become difficult to find in France. It is fairly common in the U.K. where it has never been used to flavour alcohol but used to be strewn around in houses to keep flies away.)

Put in a receptacle a coffeespoonful of wormwood leaves and flowers, pour on a litre of boiling water, stir well, cover and leave to infuse for ten minutes. Take a cupful of this infusion before each of the three main meals.

Angelica: take a tablespoonful of angelica wine (preparation No. 9) before each of the three main meals. If preferred take a coffeecupful of angelica infusion (preparation No. 7).

Salt baths: take every morning for one week in the month a bath in which a kilo of rock salt has been dissolved.

Carrots: drink for a week in each month a glass of carrot juice before each of the two main meals.

Chervil: In spring drink for one month first thing in the morning a coffeecupful of chervil juice.

Watercress: take daily for one month half an hour before the main meals a tablespoonful of watercress juice.

Walnut: drink a cupful of an infusion of walnut leaves (preparation No. 115) before each of the three main meals.

Nettles: drink four cupfuls of stinging nettle decoction daily (preparation No. 123).

Horsetail: drink a cupful of horsetail infusion first thing in the morning and last thing at night (preparation No. 131).

Tomatoes: take daily, for one month, before each of the main meals a glass of tomato juice mixed with an equal amount of celery juice.

GONORRHOEA

If gonorrhoea has been contracted a doctor should be consulted at once. Out of interest, however, here are some popular medicine suggestions for treatment of which the efficacy has not been proven. It is better to remember that prevention is better than cure.

Pellitory-of-the-wall infusion

Drink first thing in the morning a large cupful of pellitory-of-the-wall infusion (preparation No. 125).

Parsley juice

Take a coffeespoonful of fresh parsley juice first thing each morning.

Dandelion

Take with breakfast each morning a small plateful of dandelion leaves cooked in wine vinegar.

CANCER

Obviously it is unwise to trust to any popular medical procedures for the treatment of an illness as serious as cancer. However, no harm can be done if in addition to orthodox medical treatment use is also made of the infusions which popular medicine believes to be helpful.

It is said that the growth of some cancers is slowed down by drinking an infusion of periwinkle prepared in the following manner: put in a receptacle four tablespoonfuls of periwinkle leaves, pour on a litre of boiling water, stir well, cover and leave to infuse for ten minutes. Drink three cupfuls a day: one first thing in the morning, a second between breakfast and the midday meal and a third between the midday meal and the evening meal.

Similarly, an infusion of greater celandine is supposed to have the same properties (preparation No. 54a). Take four cupfuls each day: one first thing in the morning, a second between breakfast and the midday meal, a third between the midday meal and evening meal and a fourth before retiring. *(Translator's note:* greater celandine is one example – among many – of a remedy to be used with great care as it is extremely poisonous. It is also liable to confusion with the lesser celandine.

Please check the translator's notes under Nos. 54 and 54a in the Preparations Section.)

Popular medicine considers tarragon to have some value as a preventive measure if taken as an infusion for ten days in the month. A tarragon infusion is prepared as follows: put in a saucepan three tablespoonfuls of tarragon and pour on a litre of boiling water. Stir well, cover and leave to infuse for ten minutes. Take a cupful after each of the three main meals.

CELLULITE

Ivy compress

Put in a saucepan 100 g of fresh common ivy leaves to a litre of cold water. Bring slowly to the boil, leave on the boil for a quarter of an hour and, when the preparation has cooled down a little, strain through a cloth, taking care to press the leaves well while doing so. Warm up the liquid and soak compresses with it and apply them to the affected areas.

Burdock

Obtain some fresh burdock leaves. Prepare a suitable number of towels and set some water to boil. Apply the outside of the burdock leaves to the cellulite, covering with towels that have been soaked in the boiling water and well wrung out. Keep in place as long as the towels are still fairly warm. Follow the procedure twice a day for at least one week.

Seaweed

Put in a receptacle five large teaspoonfuls of dried seaweed that has been cut into small pieces together with ten tablespoonfuls of bran. Mix with hot water to obtain a reasonably liquid paste. Spread the paste on the areas of cellulite. Hold in place for twenty minutes and then wash with lukewarm water. Apply this treatment every evening for a fortnight.

Sundry methods

Footbath: take a tepid footbath for a quarter of an hour morning and night for a fortnight.

Clematis: take a cup of clematis infusion (preparation No. 62a) before each of the main meals of the day and use clematis alcohol (preparation No 62) as a lotion on the affected areas every night.
Meadowsweet: put in a receptacle three tablespoonfuls of meadowsweet – use flowers, leaves or roots (preparation No. 137). Pour on a litre of water which has been boiled and allowed to cool slowly. Stir, cover and allow to infuse for ten minutes before straining. Drink half the liquid in the course of the morning and the other half during the afternoon.
Verbena: take a cupful of verbena decoction (preparation No. 164) after each of the three main meals.
Vine leaves: take a cupful of vine leaf decoction (preparation No. 166) after each of the three main meals.

SCROFULA

(Translator's note: the term 'scrofula' has long since disappeared from use largely due to classification of different inflammations of the neck region according to underlying pathology.)

The kings of France were reputed to have the power to cure scrofula by the laying on of hands, a power that was passed to Clovis by St Remi. It was retained by the kings of France in their quality as kings which is to say that they had to be actually and firmly on the throne to be able to exercise their gift of healing. Have the Presidents of the French Republic inherited this gift? It seems that the question has never been put to the test! *(Translator's note:* Clovis I (c. 465–511) was a Merovingian king of the Franks and founder of the united Frankish kingdom; Remi or Remigius (c. 440–533) was learned as well as saintly and was elected archbishop of Rheims when he was only nineteen. The belief was shared in England–hence the name 'king's evil'–and the last to practise the Royal touch were the Stuarts.)

When there was not a king handy the method was to soak fresh mullein leaves in hot wine and apply them to the inflammation.

TIREDNESS

The procedures mentioned hereafter are applied to asthenia and the fatigue that follows an illness or overwork, in short any state requiring what is commonly called a tonic.

Salt water bath

Take before retiring a lukewarm bath in which four kilos of rock salt have been dissolved.

Thyme cure

Take in the morning three times a week a hot bath with thyme (preparation No. 154) and soak in it for fifteen minutes. Also drink a thyme infusion (preparation No. 156) after each of the three main meals.

One can complete this cure by drinking an aperitif glass of thyme wine before lunch and supper. The wine is prepared in the following way: put in a litre bottle six tablespoonfuls of thyme; fill with a good claret and leave to macerate for two weeks, shaking the bottle twice a day. Strain before using.

Sundry methods

Heath: take three times a week a hot heath bath (preparation No. 37) and lie in it for fifteen minutes.

Carrots: take a glass of carrot juice first thing in the morning every day for a fortnight.

Watercress and spinach: extract the juice from equal amounts of watercress and spinach. Drink a glass of the juice at breakfast every morning for a fortnight.

Gentian: drink a gentian infusion (preparation No. 85) twice a day: a cupful two hours before the midday meal and another one two hours before the evening meal.

Balm: drink an aperitif glass of balm wine (preparation No. 105) two hours before the midday and evening meals each day for one month.

Onion: quarter a large onion and boil it in half a litre of water until the liquid is reduced by at least a half. Leave it to macerate throughout the night. Next morning strain it and drink on an empty stomach. Follow the treatment for a fortnight.

Horseradish: drink a large cupful of horseradish decoction (preparation No. 113) with the two main meals of each day for one week.
Sage: drink half a coffeecupful of sage wine after the two main meals for one week (preparation No. 147).
Verbena: drink a cupful of verbena decoction after midday and evening meals and before retiring (preparation No. 164).

FEVER

The following methods are recommended to 'bring down' a fever.

One should not be unduly alarmed by a sudden high temperature and relief by popular medicine methods may be safely employed. If, however, the temperature is unusually high or if the fever is stubbornly recurrent a doctor ***must*** be consulted even though some measure of relief has been obtained through home medication.

Onion poultice

Find two small sacks or bags and half fill each one with chopped onions. Place the patient's feet in the bags, the tops of which should be closely tied above the ankles. This method induces profuse sweating and a subsequent fall in body temperature.

Cask or barrel method

This method is no longer praticable under present-day conditions as it was developed in the past when ways of life were different. Nevertheless, it is worth describing because it enjoyed a great reputation.

A cask or barrel large enough for the patient to sit in was the first requisite. The bottom of the barrel was spread with a thick layer of freshly cooked ivy leaves over which several litres of boiling red wine had been poured. A stool or chair on which the patient could sit was placed inside the barrel which was then covered with a blanket in such a way that only the patient's head was exposed to the air.

It is said that this method produced excellent results.

Wet sheet method

Spread a blanket on the bed and cover it with a waterproof sheet. Soak a sheet in cold water, wring it out and put it on top of the waterproof sheet. Lay the undressed patient on the wet sheet and wrap it over his whole body with the exception of his head. Place a blanket over him and pack around his body hot-water bottles to ensure that he is kept as warm as possible.

This method is said to bring about instant sweating and a sensation of relief. After half an hour to an hour remove the waterproof sheet, the damp sheet and the blanket, rub down the patient briskly and put him to bed in the normal way.

Sundry methods

Garlic: Chewing two or three cloves of garlic in the morning is said to be beneficial if one has woken up with a slight temperature.
Basil: take two or three mouthfuls of a cold infusion of basil every hour (preparation No. 22).
Borage: drink at will a borage infusion (preparation No. 36).
Camomile: follow preparation No. 44 but ensure that twelve flower heads of camomile are used instead of four.
Lettuce: prepare a lettuce decoction in the following manner: put in a saucepan two large chopped lettuce hearts to a litre of cold water. Bring slowly to the boil, simmer for ten minutes and then strain well through a fine cloth. Take a cupful of this decoction every two hours.
Meadowsweet: drink a small aperitif glass of meadowsweet wine every two hours (preparation No. 138).
Sage: if feverish on waking chew immediately some fresh sage leaves.
Verbena: take a cupful of verbena decoction (preparation No. 164) every three hours.
Violets: take a cupful of violet flower decoction every two hours (preparation No. 167).

TYPHOID FEVER

If ever there is the slightest suspicion that typhoid fever might have been contracted a doctor *must* be called immediately. The popular medicine treatment described below is only a first-aid measure to be used if there is a delay in the arrival of medical care.

Grate some raw onions into a mash and add several grated garlic cloves and some chopped nettle leaves. Spread this preparation on two towels and wrap them around the patient's feet so that the mash is packed tightly against the feet. Keep the poultice in place with a bandage and renew the treatment hourly until the doctor's arrival.

GOITRE

Goitre is provoked by the enlargement of the thyroid gland. Popular medicine has not much to offer in the way of treatment but various methods are set out below. *(Translator's note:* the treatment of goitre by orthodox medicine has advanced rapidly in recent years.)

Watercress cure

In popular medicine watercress is considered the specific for goitre. It is recommended that goitre sufferers start the two main meals of the day with a watercress salad seasoned with lemon juice. Also, according to popular medicine, a goitre sufferer should avoid eating cabbage and abstain from coffee, alcohol and tobacco.

Wine for goitre sufferers

Burn separately and reduce to ashes the following: (i) thick brown wrapping paper; (ii) rose bush bark; and (iii) natural sponge.

Put 30 g of each kind of ash on to a square of cloth; bring the four corners together and tie together to form a sachet. Place this sachet in a receptacle with a litre of white wine. Cover and leave to macerate for twenty-four hours, moving the sachet around from time to time with a wooden spoon. After maceration filter the wine and drink one liqueur glass in the morning and another in the evening every day for one month.

According to popular tradition this cure should be begun on the first day of the moon's last quarter in each month.

Ash method

Heat slowly in a frying-pan some charcoal together with an equal amount of rock salt. Put the mixture in a stocking, tie the stocking around the neck and keep it there all night.

DROPSY

Dropsy is caused by an accumulation of fluid in the body, particularly in the abdomen. The illness was far more widespread in the past than it is today and was therefore often treated at home, which gives the methods an additional interest.

Onion cure

The onion is considered in popular medicine to be the specific for dropsy. People with dropsy were advised to eat ten raw onions daily for ten days in each month. In particularly stubborn cases the only nourishment taken was milk soup (bread and milk) three times a day – morning, noon and evening. To the soup was added a large raw chopped onion.

Olive oil massage

Massage the abdomen gently with warm olive oil for a quarter of an hour early in the morning and before going to bed.

Artichoke wine

Extract the juice (preferably with a mixer) from enough artichoke leaves to produce an appreciable amount. Take care to use the leaves and not the bracts – often called 'leaves' – of the edible top of the plant. Add to the juice obtained the same amount of Madeira and bottle. Take three tablespoonfuls of this wine first thing in the morning and three more at bedtime. Always shake the bottle well before use.

Sundry methods

Birch: drink two aperitif glasses daily of birch leaf wine (preparation No. 33): a glass after breakfast and another before supper.

Follow the treatment for fifteen consecutive days.
Clematis: prepare an infusion of clematis leaves as follows: put in a receptacle a heaped tablespoonful of clematis leaves; pour a litre of boiling water on, stir, cover and let it infuse for ten minutes before straining. Drink a glass of this infusion, lightly sweetened, before each of the three main meals.
Broom: take a cupful of broom infusion (preparation No. 84) before the three main meals for one week. Renew the treatment each month.
Meadowsweet: take three cupfuls of meadowsweet infusion (preparation No. 137) one hour before the three main meals and continue daily for a fortnight.

IMPOTENCE

According to popular medicine cow parsnip (or hogweed) has the property of restoring lost virility.

Drink either an aperitif glass of cow parsnip (preparation No. 30) one hour before the two main meals or take an infusion (preparation No. 29) after the three main meals.

WENS

Parsley poultice

Pound firmly in a mortar a sprig of parsley leaves and the same amount of fresh chervil leaves – about a cupful of each – and add little by little half a coffeespoonful of table salt and a tablespoonful of olive oil.

Wrap this preparation in a piece of gauze and apply it to the wen. Hold in place with a dressing. Renew the treatment morning and night, keeping the morning poultice all day and that of the evening all night, and persist with it until there is a noticeable improvement when only the poultice at night will be necessary until the complete disappearance of the wen.

MENINGITIS

Call a doctor immediately at the first signs of meningitis. *(Translator's note:* it should be stressed that meningitis characterized by a violent headache, temperature and stiff neck can kill in a matter of hours if medical help is not sought.) However, if in desperate straits, one can fall back on the only two popular medicine methods that have been handed down to us.

Cabbage leaf application

Cover the patient's head completely, in the form of a helmet, with several layers of cabbage leaves (preparation No. 55) held in place by a towel and left until the doctor's arrival.

Onion bath

Fill two sacks with finely-chopped onions. Put each of the patient's feet into a sack so that the onion is packed around them. Tie the mouths of the sacks closely above the ankles and leave in place until medical aid arrives.

MALARIA

Now that sophisticated medication is available such as chloroquine and related substances – the methods used in popular medicine are of mostly academic interest. But if no modern drug were available it is recommended that the patient drink a cup of coffee to which an equal quantity of hot water and the juice of a lemon have been added.

SPLEEN DISORDERS

Popular medicine has only one remedy to offer for spleen disorders and that is syrup of asparagus tips (preparation No. 18).

Take a tablespoonful of this syrup before the three main meals.

EXCESSIVE PERSPIRATION

According to popular tradition sage has the ability to check excessive sweating.

Drink one cupful of sage infusion (preparation No. 145) last thing at night for one week. During the following week drink a cupful every other day and if the result is satisfactory reduce the dosage still further to a cupful once every three days. Another method is to take a tablespoonful of sage wine (preparation No. 147) after the two main meals of the day for a fortnight.

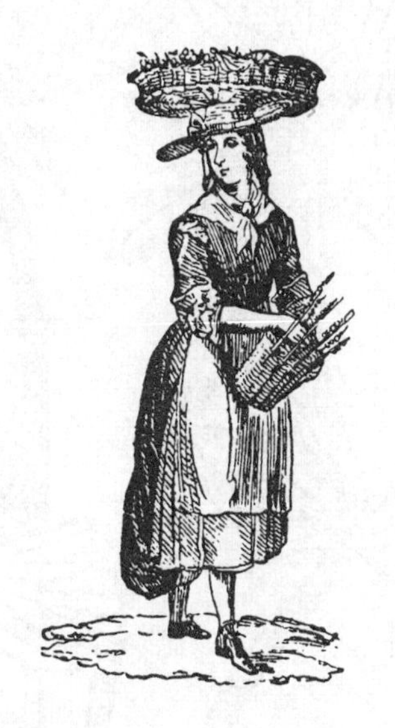

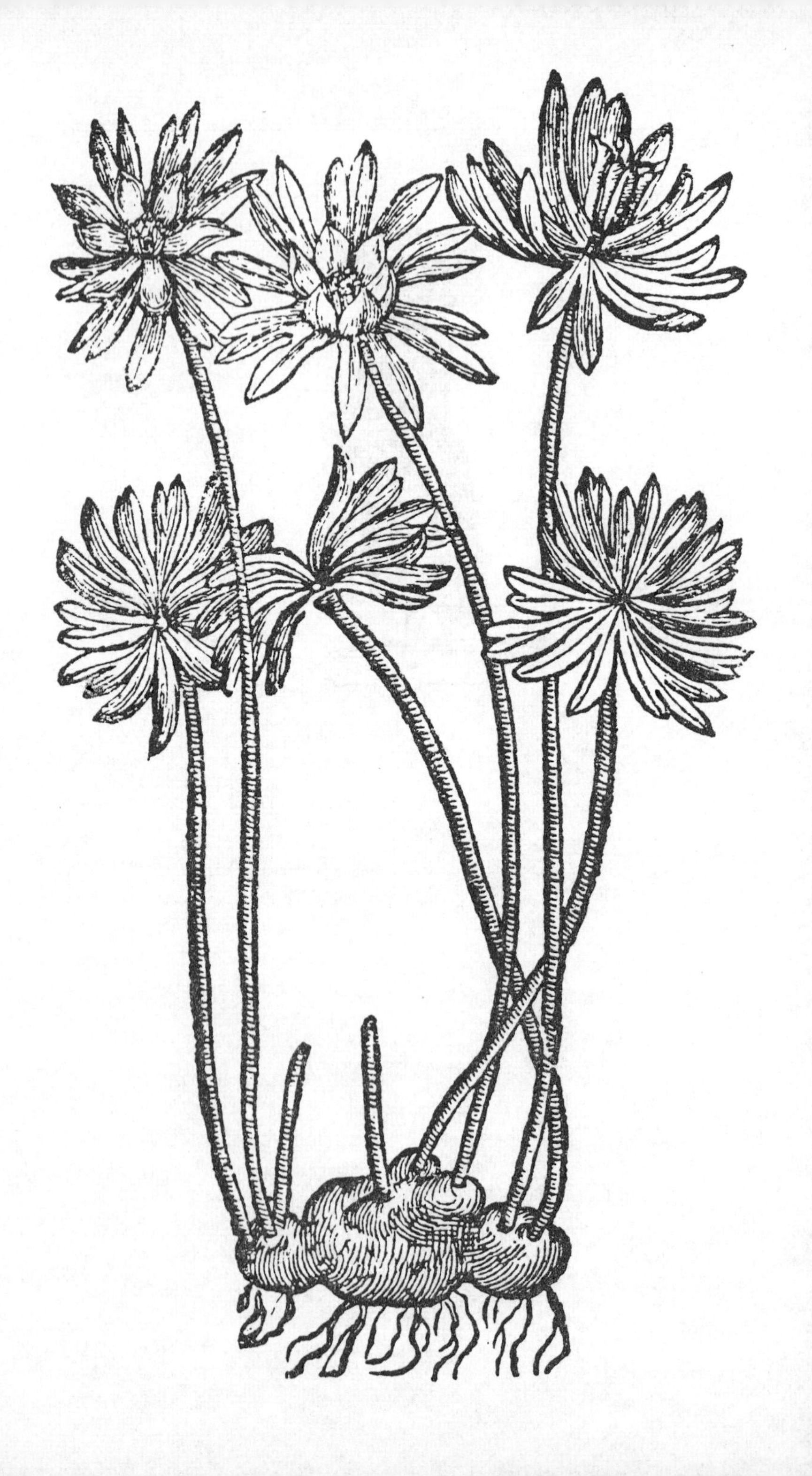

Nervous System and Mental Disorders

INSOMNIA · MIGRAINES · SHYNESS · HYSTERIA
NERVOUS EXCITABILITY · TENDENCY TO ANXIETY
TENDENCY TO NEURASTHENIA · NEUROSIS

INSOMNIA

Insomnia is nowadays a common affliction and the use of sleeping pills more often than not only aggravates the condition. Therefore popular medicine can be particularly useful in this field. Insomnia is treated mostly by infusions, certain of which work well with some people but not with others. Try a variety of methods, therefore, until you find the one that suits you. They are also applicable to cases of broken sleep and a tendency to nightmares.

General rules for sound sleep

According to popular traditions a few general rules have to be respected before one can hope to obtain sound sleep. You should sleep with the window open; use a hard mattress, preferably made of horsehair; and place your bed so that your head is to the north and your feet face southwards.

Those prone to insomnia are also advised to watch the food eaten at evening meals and should eat either corn salad (lamb's lettuce) seasoned with the juice of a lemon and a little garlic or cooked lettuce.

A procedure said to help one to fall asleep easily is to massage the entire body with a horsehair glove, take a brisk cold shower and go to bed without drying oneself.

An 'arm bath' is also advised. Fill the basin with cold water and soak in it the folded arms, elbows resting on the bottom, for ten seconds. Put on a pyjama jacket and go to bed without drying the arms.

Sundry methods
Rose hip: take a large cupful of unsweetened rose hip decoction before retiring (preparation No. 72).
Quince: take a small coffeecupful of quince leaf infusion before retiring (preparation No. 63).
Poppy: drink, one hour after each of the main meals, a cupful of an infusion of poppy petals (preparation No. 65).
Hawthorn: drink, before retiring, a teacupful of an infusion of hawthorn flowers (preparation No. 19).
Almonds: drink a teacupful of a decoction of almond shells (preparation No. 5) late in the afternoon and another one at bedtime.
Melilot: take an hour after each of the main meals a teacupful of melilot infusion (preparation No. 103), lukewarm and well sweetened.
Saffron: put in a mug 2 g of saffron: fill with boiling water, cover with a saucer, leave to infuse for ten minutes. Take this preparation, unsweetened, before going to bed.
Lettuce: take one hour after the evening meal a lettuce decoction (preparation No. 93).
Valerian: drink before retiring a large cupful of valerian infusion slightly sweetened (preparation No. 160). If possible take also, a little earlier, a bath with a valerian preparation (preparation No. 160a).
Hawthorn tincture: before retiring, drink a small glass of a good sweet wine with a tablespoonful of hawthorn tincture in it (preparation No. 20).
Mullein: drink before retiring a cupful of mullein infusion (preparation No. 31).
Balm: drink a cupful of balm infusion, slightly sweetened, after each meal (preparation No. 104).
Orange leaf: take before retiring a large cupful of an infusion of orange leaves or flowers (preparation No. 119).
Lime (Linden): before retiring, drink a large cup of slightly-sweetened lime infusion (preparation No. 158).
Rosemary: put in a litre bottle six tablespoonfuls of rosemary cut into small pieces. Fill the bottle with a good red wine, cork and leave to macerate for one week, shaking the bottle each day. At

the end of the week strain and add ten lumps of sugar. Take a glass of this preparation before retiring.

Rosemary infusion (preparation No. 140) can also be drunk one hour after the evening meal.

Aniseed: take after supper a spoonful of aniseed, chew and keep in the mouth as long as possible.

MIGRAINES

In the past migraine was a very common complaint, particularly among women, and every family had its secret remedy for it. Most of the methods which have been handed down to us have some effect but, as is always the case in popular medicine, what works with one person often has no effect on another. That is why, yet again, it is often necessary to try several remedies before hitting on the right one.

Vinegar inhalations

Fill two-thirds of a receptacle with boiling water (an earthenware jug should be used) and add a full glass of vinegar. Cover head and shoulders with a thick towel and inhale the preparation for a quarter of an hour. Thoroughly dry the face and lie down for half an hour.

Pepper poultice

Mix powdered pepper, i.e. ground very fine, with *eau de vie* to form a thick paste. Apply a strip of this paste across the forehead and lie down until there is a marked improvement. It is said that while doing so one should recite three Pater Nosters and three Ave Marias. For some it is enough to lie down for half an hour while trying, at the same time, to banish one's daily preoccupations from the mind. (*Translator's note:* nowadays one might consider transcendental meditation or yoga in this context.)

White of egg poultice

Beat until very firm three whites of egg, adding as you do so a quarter of a coffeespoonful of saffron. Wrap the mixture in a gauze and apply to the forehead. Lie down with the eyes closed until the pain diminishes.

Ivy wine

Pound in a mortar a good handful of ivy leaves and the same quantity of mugwort leaves. Put the mixture in a receptacle; add a litre and a half of white wine; cover and leave to macerate for four days, stirring with a wooden spoon twice a day. After this time strain and bottle.

This wine is recommended for chronic sufferers from migraine. An aperitif glass of wine is taken on an empty stomach in the morning and breakfast should not be eaten until two hours later.

Compresses

Prepare two receptacles: one with very hot water to which a glass of vinegar has been added, the other filled with very cold water. Soak the towel in the hot water, wring it out and apply it to the patient's stomach; soak another towel in the cold water and apply it to the nape of the neck.

Renew with new compresses every five minutes until relief is obtained.

Sundry methods

Almonds: at the first indication of migraine drink a cupful of almond shell decoction (preparation No. 5). One can also pound bitter almonds and apply them to the forehead.

Angelica: when the pain of migraine starts, take a coffeespoonful of angelica tincture in a little water (preparation No. 8). If the migraines are chronic take a coffeespoonful of the same preparation after each of the three main meals for a week.

Lemon: drink a cup of very strong and unsweetened coffee to which has been added the juice of half a lemon.

Cherries: crush some cherries after having removed the stones. Enclose the fruit in gauze and apply to the forehead. Lie down until there is marked relief.

Cabbage: apply a cabbage leaf poultice to the forehead (preparation No. 55). Lie down for half an hour.

Balm: to combat chronic migraine drink a cupful of balm infusion (preparation No. 104) after the two main meals.

Mint: a cupful of mint infusion (preparation No. 106) can relieve migraine.

Walnut leaves: take a footbath to the water of which has been added an infusion of walnut leaves (preparation No. 115). Keep the feet in the bath for fifteen minutes.
Onions: peel and slice a large raw onion, taking care to inhale the aroma. Raw onion slices can also be applied to the forehead and kept there until the irritation becomes unbearable.
Potatoes: grate some raw potatoes and make a poultice with the pulp which is then applied to the forehead. Lie down for half an hour.
Horseradish: grate some unpeeled horseradish. Make a poultice with the pulp and apply to the forehead. Lie down and leave the poultice in place for an hour.
Lime (linden): a cupful of lime decoction (preparation No. 158) taken after the three main meals is sometimes helpful to migraine sufferers.
Valerian: drink a cupful of valerian infusion (preparation No. 160) before the three main meals.
Veronica: at the first signs of migraine take a cupful of unsweetened veronica infusion (preparation No. 162).
Verbena: soak a cloth with verbena decoction (preparation No. 164) and apply to the forehead. Lie down for a quarter of an hour and then drink a cupful of verbena infusion (preparation No. 165).
Violets: drink during the day five cupfuls of violet decoction (preparation No. 167).

SHYNESS

According to popular traditions the following preparation gives particularly shy or emotional persons self-assurance when it is needed, e.g. when making a speech or attending an important interview.

Put in a small saucepan a liqueur glass of rum and an aperitif glass of orange flowers. Heat over a low flame and when boiling point has been reached toss at once into the liquid a tablespoonful of lime (linden) flowers, half a coffeespoonful of tea and six camomile heads. Remove immediately from the heat, cover and allow to infuse for half an hour. Strain, pressing the leaves well, and allow to cool before use.

HYSTERIA

According to popular tradition, someone bordering on an attack will be calmed down upon strongly inhaling a sliced onion.

NERVOUS EXCITABILITY

Lime (linden) bath

Take a lime bath (preparation No. 159) just before the evening meal.

Walnut bath

Put in a large receptacle 400 g of walnut leaves to three litres of cold water. Bring to the boil, boil for a quarter of an hour and strain. Add this decoction to the water of a hot bath to be taken before retiring.

Valerian bath

Before going to bed take a bath to which valerian has been added (preparation No. 160a).

Savory bath

Put in a receptacle 300 g of flowering tips of savory. Pour on two litres of boiling water, cover and leave to infuse for ten minutes and strain. Add this preparation to the hot water of a bath.

Sundry methods

Quince leaves: take a half-cupful of quince infusion (preparation No. 63).
Lavender: drink between meals two cupfuls of lavender flower infusion daily (preparation No. 94a).
Balm: take one cupful of balm infusion (preparation No. 104) after each of the three main meals.

Lily-of-the-valley: drink first thing in the morning and last thing at night a cupful of lily-of-the-valley infusion (preparation No. 111).
Orange leaves: drink after the three main meals a cupful of orange leaf infusion (preparation No. 119).
Valerian: drink before retiring two cupfuls of valerian infusion (preparation No. 160).

TENDENCY TO ANXIETY

In popular medicine the following infusions are said to help those who are prone to anxiety.

Bird's-foot trefoil infusion
Take a cupful of bird's-foot trefoil infusion (preparation No. 98) after each of the main meals of the day for ten days of the month.
Rose hip decoction
Drink a litre of the decoction (preparation No. 72) throughout the day.
Basil infusion
Drink one cupful of basil infusion (preparation No. 22) after each of the three main meals.

TENDENCY TO NEURASTHENIA

Popular medicine recommends the following infusions for the treatment of depression and neurasthenia.

Borage infusion
Drink three cupfuls daily between meals (preparation No. 36).

Rhubarb infusion
Drink one cupful before the three main meals (preparation No. 139).

Sage infusion
Drink one cupful after each of the three main meals (preparation No. 145).

Willow infusion
Three cupfuls to be taken daily: one on an empty stomach, one after lunch and the third after supper (preparation No. 148).

Tansy infusion
Drink three cupfuls daily between meals (preparation No. 153).

Veronica decoction
Take one cupful half an hour before the three main meals (preparation No. 161).

NEUROSIS

Popular medicine believes that neuroses, and particularly obsessions, being afflictions of the mind, can only respond to treatment by the mind. Two daily readings from the Bible are recommended: Psalm 72 and Chapter 1 of the Gospel according to St John. Is this merely a superstition? Or are certain words capable of exerting a spiritual influence?

At the same time, however, popular medicine suggests that those who are prey to neuroses should drink a glass of watercress juice before breakfast or take before each of the main meals of the day half a coffeecupful of tincture of angelica (preparation No. 8). Futhermore, they are advised to wear, or to hang in the bedroom, a St Benedict medallion.

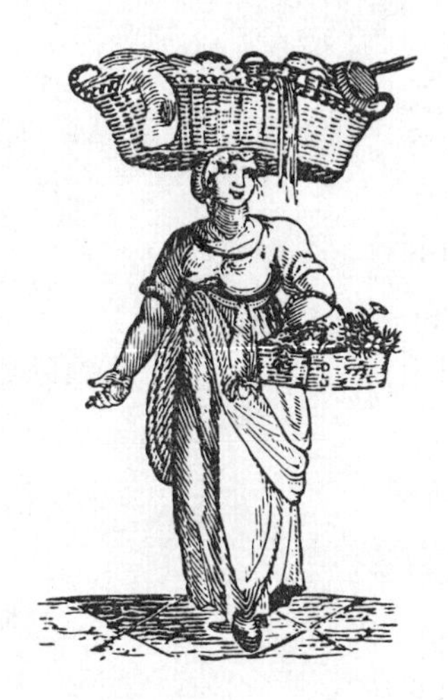

Part Two

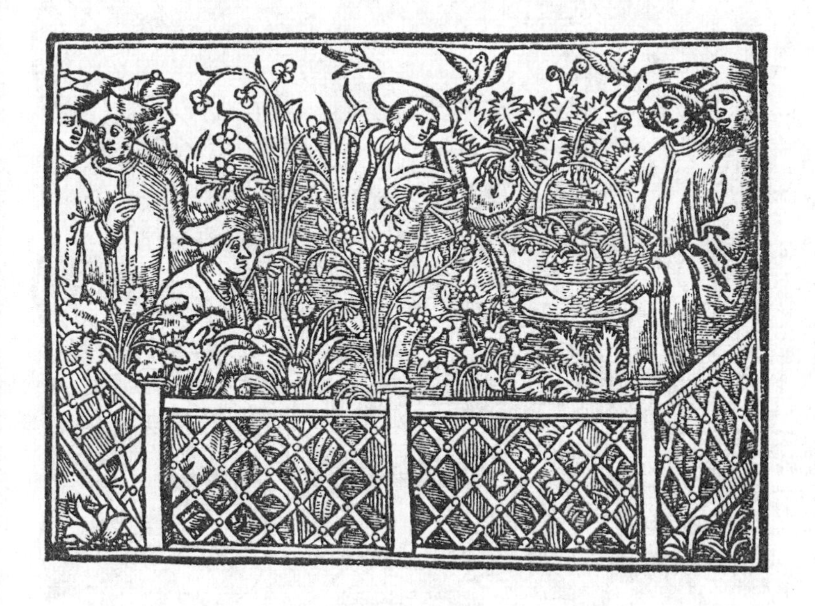

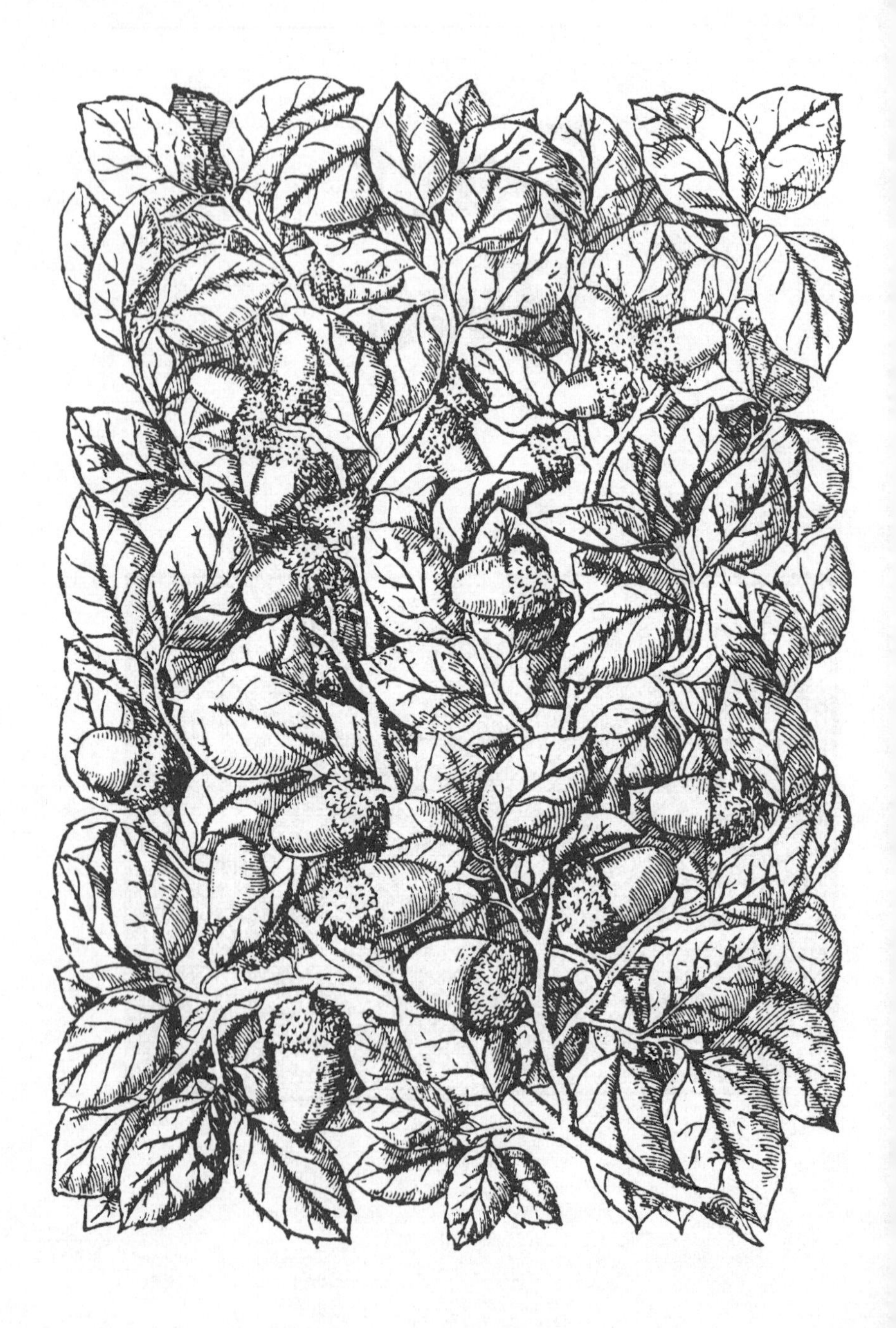

The Preparations

The majority of the preparations listed here are derived from herbs. It must be emphasized that plants should not be picked haphazardly by amateurs if intended for medicinal use. Herbs that are to be used in these preparations must only be gathered under favourable conditions. Moreover, if they are to retain curative properties or, in certain cases, to lose toxic elements, they must undergo certain treatments,

(*Translator's note:* the author goes on to say, in the French edition, that the profession of herbalist was suppressed in France in 1945 and that most herbs can now be bought only in pharmacies. This is not the case in the U.K. where there is a National Institute of Medical Herbalists whose members are qualified herbal practitioners and there are many herbalists who prepare and sell herbs over the counter and by post.

The British have always shown greater interest in plant studies, birdwatching and country life in general than the French have. At the time when Gilbert White was writing his *Natural History of Selborne* his near contemporary Jean-Jacques Rousseau was being caricatured and mocked for his botanizing. Many people in Britain are familiar with the Latin names of plants which are essential to accurate identification. For that reason I have added them to the common English names in the headings of the preparations.

Few will come to harm through using a cabbage leaf poultice, an infusion of fennel or dog rose hip wine, and many of the herbs mentioned here may be gathered and used without mishap. Remember to check the amounts and proportions, to follow the directions and adhere strictly to the recommended dosage. Where there is the slightest doubt as to a herb's identity, provenance or suitable condition, discard it and rely on the herbalist's stock.)

PREPARATION NO. 1

Infusion of Agrimony *(Agrimonia eupatoria)*

Principal indication: hoarseness

Put in a container a handful of agrimony leaves that have been lightly crushed between the hands. Pour on a litre of boiling water and stir until well mixed. Cover the receptacle and infuse for ten minutes. Strain, and when needed heat the quantity of liquid required, taking care not to let it boil. Sweeten the infusion, preferably with honey.

PREPARATION NO. 2

Alcoholature of Garlic *(Alium sativum)*

Principal indication: high blood pressure

Crush thoroughly 150 g of garlic and macerate in a litre of 40° *eau de vie* for six weeks. Strain and store in a bottle. For immediate use one can extract the juice of 500 g of garlic to which an equal quantity of alcohol at 40° is added.

PREPARATION NO. 3

Infusion of Lady's Mantle *(Alchemilla filicaulis)*

Principal indications: post-miscarriage complications; leucorrhoea

Put two tablespoonfuls of crushed lady's mantle leaves into a receptacle. Pour on half a litre of boiling water, shake well, cover and leave to infuse for ten minutes before straining.

PREPARATION NO. 4

Decoction of Lady's Mantle

Principal indication: pruritis

Put 50 g of crushed lady's mantle leaves into a saucepan. Pour on a litre of cold water. Cover and heat gently up to boiling point. Allow to boil for ten minutes then strain at once.

PREPARATION NO. 5

Decoction of Almond Shells *(Amygdalus communis)*

Principal indications: insomnia; headaches

Put two tablespoonfuls of coarsely-crushed almond shells into a saucepan with half a litre of cold water. Cover and bring slowly to the boil. Boil for ten minutes and strain immediately.

PREPARATION NO. 6

Milk of Almonds

Principal indication: stomach ache

First prepare a lettuce infusion in the following way: cut up 50 g of large lettuce leaves (preferably from a mature lettuce). Put the pieces into a receptacle and add a litre of boiling water, stirring well. Cover and leave to infuse for ten minutes. Strain. While the lettuce infusion is cooling shell thirty almonds and peel them. To facilitate the removal of the skins plunge the almonds into boiling water for a few minutes. Pound them in a mortar, adding from time to time a little water and some granulated sugar (about three lumps, well crushed). When a fine paste is obtained stir slowly into it the lettuce infusion then strain through a piece of fine muslin.

PREPARATION NO. 7

Infusion of Angelica *(Angelica archangelica)*

Principal indications: anaemia and indigestion

Take two heaped tablespoonfuls of finely-chopped fresh angelica root or stems (if fresh angelica is not available, candied angelica can be used). Put in a receptacle and add a litre of boiling water. Cover and allow to infuse for twenty minutes before straining.

PREPARATION NO. 8

Angelica Tincture

Principal indications: depression; headaches

Chop finely 100 g of fresh angelica root. Put in a receptacle with a decilitre of *eau-de-vie* at 90°. Cover and leave to macerate in a warm place for four days. Then strain, making sure that all the liquid is squeezed from the roots. Store in a bottle.

PREPARATION NO. 9

Angelica Wine

Principal indications: anaemia; stomach cramp

Put in a litre bottle 50 g of finely-chopped fresh angelica root, 4 g of crushed cinnamon, and fill the bottle with Malaga. Cork the bottle and leave to macerate for four days before filtering.

PREPARATION NO. 10

Decoction of Wormwood *(Artemisia absinthium)*

Principal indications: stomach pains; bowel pains; excessively light periods

Toss into a litre of boiling water three dessertspoonfuls of aniseed (if seeds are not available use wormwood leaves instead). Leave to boil for two minutes. Cover and let it infuse for ten minutes. Strain the preparation.

PREPARATION NO. 11

Wormwood Cordial

Principal indication: aerophagia

Crush thoroughly 50 g of aniseed. Put in a litre bottle with 1 g of cinnamon and 300 g of granulated sugar. Fill the bottle with *eau de vie* at 40°. Put the well-stoppered bottle in a dark place and leave the mixture to macerate for six weeks. At the end of this time filter the preparation.

PREPARATION NO. 12

Infusion of Wormwood, Caraway and Cumin *(Artemisia absinthium, Carum carui, Cummin cynenum)*

Principal indication: aerophagia

Toss into a litre of boiling water a tablespoonful of aniseed, a tablespoonful of cumin seed and two tablespoonfuls of caraway seed. Stir well, cover and leave to infuse for ten minutes before straining.

PREPARATION NO. 13

Infusion of Mugwort *(Artemisia vulgaris)*

Principal indications: irregular and interrupted periods

Put in a receptacle three dessertspoonfuls of crushed mugwort leaves (or a mixture of leaves and flowers). Stir, cover and leave to infuse for ten minutes before straining. It is preferable not to sweeten the infusion.

PREPARATION NO. 14

Infusion of Mugwort and Shepherd's Purse *(Artemisia vulgaris, Thlaspi bursa pastoris)*

Principal indication: painful periods

Place in a saucepan a generous tablespoonful of mugwort leaves and a tablespoonful of shepherd's purse flowers and leaves. Pour on half a litre of cold water, bring slowly to the boil, keeping a lid on the saucepan. Allow to boil for three minutes before straining.

PREPARATION NO. 15

Decoction of Artichoke *(Cynara scolymus)*

Principal indications: arthritis, biliousness

Cut into pieces four fresh artichoke leaves (they must be the plant's actual leaves, not the bracts surrounding the part that is eaten). Put the leaves in a saucepan to a litre of cold water. Cover and bring to the boil. Allow the leaves to boil slowly for a quarter of an hour before straining.

PREPARATION NO. 16

Maceration of Artichoke

Principal indications: diarrhoea; rheumatism

Cut into small pieces 200 g of fresh artichoke leaves or, better still, 100 g of chopped artichoke root if available added to 100 g of chopped leaves. Place roots and leaves in a bowl with a litre of white wine. Cover and leave to macerate for a week. Strain through a fine cloth and store in a bottle.

PREPARATION NO. 17

Artichoke Wine

Principal indications: bilious attacks

Cut into small pieces 40 g of fresh artichoke leaves and put them into a litre bottle. Fill the bottle with white wine and leave to macerate for a week, shaking the bottle once or twice a day. Strain the preparation and transfer to another bottle.

PREPARATION NO. 18

Asparagus Syrup *(Asparagus officinalis)*

Principal indications: enlarged spleen; palpitations

Cut a pound of tips from some asparagus; crush them or put them through a mixer. Weigh the juice thus obtained and add to it twice its weight in sugar, preferably cane sugar. Dissolve the sugar in the asparagus juice in a *bain marie* and heat it to a syrupy consistency. Allow the preparation to cool and pour it into bottles which are then well sealed. (It is better to use several small bottles rather than one large one.) Store in a cool place.

PREPARATION NO. 19

Infusion of Hawthorn *(Crataegus oxyeantha)*

Principal indications: heart conditions; high blood pressure; insomnia; painful periods

Place in a receptacle four tablespoonfuls of hawthorn flowers. Pour on a litre of boiling water. Stir well, cover and allow to infuse for ten minutes before straining.

If this infusion is prescribed for the treatment of painful menstruation leave it to infuse for a further ten minutes.

PREPARATION NO. 20

Tincture of Hawthorn

Principal indications: anxiety; high blood pressure; insomnia

Quarter fill a litre bottle with hawthorn flowers (rather less than more). Top up with *eau de vie,* cork tightly and leave to macerate for two weeks, shaking the bottle once a day. Then transfer to another bottle through a filter.

PREPARATION NO. 21

Decoction of Burdock *(Arctium lappa)*

Principal indications: acne; dartres

Place in a saucepan 50 g of burdock roots which have been cut up into small pieces. Add half a litre of cold water and bring slowly to the boil. Boil for a quarter of an hour before straining.

PREPARATION NO. 22

Infusion of Basil *(Ocimum basilicum)*

Principal indications: colic; throat infections; neurasthenia
Place in a receptacle five tablespoonfuls of basil that has been cut into small pieces. (Use either the whole of the plant or just the flowers.) Pour on a litre of boiling water. Stir, cover and leave to infuse for a quarter of an hour before filtering. If the preparation is used to treat colic it is better administered unsweetened.

PREPARATION NO. 23

Decoction of Crane's Bill *(Geranium robertanium)*

Principal indication: aphthas (mouth ulcers)
Place in a saucepan a handful of crane's bill to a third of a litre of cold water. Bring slowly to the boil. Boil for five minutes and filter.

PREPARATION NO. 24

Decoction of Wood Avens or Herb Bennet *(Geum urganum)*

Place in a saucepan five tablespoonfuls of dried wood avens to half a litre of cold water. Leave to soak for an hour before bringing slowly to the boil. Bring to the boil several times and strain. This decoction should be prepared in an enamel saucepan.

PREPARATION NO. 25

Tincture of Wood Avens Roots

Crush with a bottle or rolling pin 100 g of dried wood avens root. Place in a litre bottle and top with *eau de vie* at 60°. Leave to macerate for two weeks, shaking the bottle once a day. Filter the preparation.

PREPARATION NO. 26

Infusion of Cornflower *(Centaurea cyanus)*

Place in a receptacle four tablespoonfuls of cornflower blooms. Pour on a litre of boiling water. Cover and leave to infuse for twenty minutes. Strain.

PREPARATION NO. 27

Decoction of Cornflower

Principal indications: aphthas; inflammation of the eyelid; thrush; halitosis

Put in a saucepan two tablespoonfuls of cornflower blooms to a litre of cold water. Cover and bring slowly to the boil. Boil for a quarter of an hour. Allow the preparation to cool before filtering.

PREPARATION NO. 28

Cornflower Wine

Principal indications: gout; rheumatism

Put in a litre bottle six tablespoonfuls of cornflower blooms. Fill the bottle with claret, seal tightly and leave to macerate for a week, shaking the bottle once a day. Filter and decant to another bottle.

PREPARATION NO. 29

Infusion of Cow Parsnip or Hogweed *(Heracleum sphondylium)*

Principal indication: impotence

Place in a receptacle two tablespoonfuls of cow parsnip roots and leaves which have been cut into small pieces. Pour on half a litre of boiling water. Stir and cover the preparation, leaving it to infuse for ten minutes. Strain.

PREPARATION NO. 30

Cow Parsnip Wine

Principal indication: impotence

Place in a litre bottle six tablespoonfuls of cow parsnip roots and leaves which have been cut into small pieces. Fill with a good red wine, seal tightly and leave to macerate for twenty-four hours, shaking the bottle from time to time. Decant through a filter. Sweeten to taste before use.

PREPARATION NO. 31

Infusion of Mullein *(Verbascum thapsus)*

Put in a receptacle three tablespoonfuls of mullein flowers. Pour on a litre of boiling water. Cover and allow to infuse for ten minutes. Meanwhile fold in two a piece of fine cloth and insert between the folds a layer of cotton wool. Strain the preparation through this to trap the mullein bristles which could irritate the mucous membranes.

PREPARATION NO. 32

Infusion of Birch Leaves *(Betula pendula)*

Principal indications: gout; rheumatism; retention of urine

Put in a receptacle five tablespoonfuls of well-crushed birch leaves. Pour on a litre of boiling water. Stir and cover and leave to infuse for a quarter of an hour. Then add a pinch of bicarbonate of soda and strain. The preparation may be sweetened to taste.

PREPARATION NO. 33

Infusion of Birch Leaves

Principal indication: dropsy

Place in a receptacle two tablespoonfuls of well-crushed birch leaves. Pour on a litre of a good red wine that has been warmed but not boiled. Cover and allow to infuse for a quarter of an hour before straining. The preparation is taken cold.

PREPARATION NO. 34

Decoction of Alder Buckthorn *(Rhamnus frangula)*

Principal indications: calculia; dartres; scabies. Alder buckthorn decoction is also a laxative suitable for people with delicate bowels

Place in a receptacle five tablespoonfuls of alder buckthorn bark to a litre of cold water.

Be sure to obtain your supply from a herbalist or chemist because the bark has to undergo a special treatment and be left to dry for at least a year. If this has not been done it could provoke painful colic and vomiting.

Cover the receptacle and bring slowly to the boil. Boil for twenty minutes and allow to infuse for four hours before straining. The infusion to be taken sweetened.

If used as a laxative, take two tablespoonfuls only of the decoction, or even less.

PREPARATION NO. 35

Decoction of Borage *(Borrago officinalis)*

Principal indications: gout; influenza; rheumatism; colds

Place in a saucepan two tablespoonfuls of dried borage (flowers, pieces of crushed twig, leaves) to half a litre of cold water. Cover and bring slowly to the boil. Boil for five minutes and allow to infuse for a quarter of an hour before straining.

PREPARATION NO. 36

Infusion of Borage

Principal indications: fever; anxiety; depression; measles; scarlet fever

Place in a receptacle two tablespoonfuls of borage flowers or three tablespoonfuls of borage leaves (flowers and leaves mixed can also be used) and pour on a litre of boiling water. Cover and leave to infuse for five minutes before straining.

PREPARATION NO. 36A

Shepherd's Purse Wine *(Thlaspi bursa pastoris)*

Principal indications: haemorrhage

This wine must be prepared with fresh shepherd's purse. Put in a receptacle 250 g of the plant, chopped into pieces, and pour on a litre of white wine. Cover and leave to macerate for a week, stirring once or twice a day. The receptacle should be placed in a warm room during the period of maceration. Then the preparation is heated slowly but not brought to the boil after which it is filtered and bottled.

PREPARATION NO. 37

Heath Baths *(Erica vulgaris)*

Principal indications: asthenia

Put in a large receptacle 500 g of chopped heath (also known as bell-heather) and add five litres of cold water. Bring to the boil and boil for about ten minutes. Strain the decoction and pour it into the hot water of a bath.

PREPARATION NO. 38

Decoction of Heath

Principal indications: cystitis; diarrhoea; nephritis; rheumatism

Put in a saucepan four tablespoonfuls of flowers and twigs of heath, cut into small pieces. Add a litre of cold water. Cover and leave to macerate for two hours. Bring slowly to the boil and simmer for five minutes.

The preparation should be allowed to settle for fifteen minutes before it is filtered.

PREPARATION NO. 39

Oil of Heath

Principal indication: rheumatism

This oil must be prepared from freshly-gathered heath. Place in a receptacle 100 g of chopped heath (the greater part should consist of the flowers). Add half a litre of olive oil. Cover the vessel and stir once a day during the maceration of one week. Then filter the preparation and bottle it.

PREPARATION NO. 40

Decoction of Heath, Strawberry-Tree Leaves and White Deadnettle *(Erica vulgaris, Arbutus unedo, Lamium album)*

Principal indication: retention of urine

Place in a receptacle six tablespoonfuls of sprigs of flowering heath, two tablespoonfuls of strawberry-tree leaves and two tablespoonfuls of chopped white deadnettle sprigs and flowers (both the white and red deadnettle are unrelated to the stinging nettle and neither stings). Add two litres of cold water, cover the receptacle, bring slowly to the boil and boil for five minutes before straining.

PREPARATION NO. 41

Decoction of Box *(Buxus sempervirens)*

Principal indications: liver diseases; skin diseases

Place in a receptacle four tablespoonfuls of dried box leaves to a litre of cold water. (Fresh box leaves can also be used but a double quantity is needed: eight or nine tablespoonfuls to a litre of water.) Cover the receptacle, bring slowly to the boil, simmer for quarter of an hour and then strain.

PREPARATION NO. 42

Infusion of Calamint *(Calamintha sylvatica)*

Principal indications: buzzing in the ears; hiccups

Place in a receptacle six tablespoonfuls of flowering tips and leaves of calamint to a litre of boiling water. Stir, cover and allow to infuse for five minutes before straining.

If the preparation prepared in this way has no effect try a stronger mixture of ten tablespoonfuls to a litre of water instead of six.

PREPARATION NO. 43

Oil of Camomile or Chamomile or Mayweed *(Matricaria chamomilla)*

Principal indications: sprains; gout; rheumatism

Place in a receptacle ten tablespoonfuls of camomile flowers to half a litre of olive oil. Heat in a *bain marie* for two hours, leave to cool, strain, taking care to press the flowers well. Filter again before bottling.

PREPARATION NO. 44

Infusion of Camomile

Principal indications: anorexia; stomach cramp; influenza; neuralgia; painful periods

Put in a receptacle four tablespoonfuls of camomile flowers and pour on a litre of boiling water. Cover and leave to infuse for ten minutes. Strain, pressing well the flowers. The infusion to be sweetened only slightly.

PREPARATION NO. 45

Camomile Infusion for external use

Principal indication: pruritis

Place in a receptacle five tablespoonfuls of camomile flowers. Pour on about two cupfuls of boiling water, stir and cover and leave to infuse for a quarter of an hour before straining, taking care to squeeze the flowers and adding a coffeespoonful of white vinegar to the preparation.

PREPARATION NO. 46

Camomile Wine

Principal indications: anorexia; prevention of indigestion

Put in a litre bottle five tablespoonfuls of camomile flowers and twenty lumps of sugar. Fill with a good white wine. Seal the bottle tightly and leave to macerate in a cool, dark place for one month, shaking the bottle once a day. Then filter and decant.

PREPARATION NO. 47

Decoction of Wild Carrot *(Daucus carota)*

Principal indications: retention of urine; eyesight troubles

Place in a saucepan four tablespoonfuls of dried wild carrot root that has been cut into small pieces. Add a litre of cold water, bring slowly to the boil. Boil for a quarter of an hour. Allow the preparation to infuse for half an hour before straining.

PREPARATION NO. 48

Decoction of Blackcurrant *(Ribes nigrum)*

Principal indication: tonsilitis

Place in a saucepan four heaped tablespoonfuls of dried blackcurrants to a litre of cold water. Bring slowly to the boil, cook for a quarter of an hour and strain.

PREPARATION NO. 49

Decoction of Blackcurrant Leaves

Principal indications: proteinuria; arthritis; cystitis; retention of urine

Soak some crumpled blackcurrant leaves four tablespoonfuls to a litre of cold water. After an hour cover the receptacle and bring slowly to the boil. Boil for one minute and leave to infuse for a quarter of an hour before straining.

PREPARATION NO. 50

Infusion of Blackcurrant Leaves

Place in a receptacle five tablespoonfuls of crumpled blackcurrant leaves. Pour on a litre of boiling water. Stir, cover the receptacle and leave to infuse for twenty minutes before straining.

PREPARATION NO. 51

Infusion of Chervil *(Anthriscus cerefolium)*

Principal indications: arteriosclerosis; biliousness; excessively light periods

Put in a receptacle 50 g of fresh chopped chervil (leaves and stems). Pour on a litre of boiling water. Stir, cover and allow to infuse for ten minutes before straining. It is preferable to leave the infusion unsweetened before drinking it.

PREPARATION NO. 52

Decoction of Cherry Stalks *(Prunus cerasus)*

Principal indications: bronchitis; calculia; renal colic; retention of urine

Put in a saucepan 100 g of either fresh or dried cherry stalks, cut into two or three pieces, to a litre of cold water. Cover and bring slowly to the boil. Boil for five minutes. Meanwhile put in another receptacle 250 g of slightly crushed cherries or two small sliced apples that have not been peeled. Pour the boiling liquid on the fruit, cover and allow to infuse for half an hour. Strain, squeezing gently the fruit.

PREPARATION NO. 53

Infusion of Cherry Leaves

Principal indication: constipation

Put in a receptacle three tablespoonfuls of crumpled cherry tree leaves. Pour on a litre of boiling water. Stir well, cover, leave to infuse for twenty minutes before straining.

PREPARATION NO. 54

Ointment of Greater Celandine *(Chelidonium majus)*

Principal indications: eczema; lupus

Chop finely 100 g of fresh greater celandine leaves and add slowly an equal weight of lard, mixing well. If no leaves are available use instead 20 g of dried root ground to a fine powder. *(Translator's note:* the greater celandine, a member of the poppy family, is not to be confused with the lesser celandine *(Ranunculus ficaria)*, a member of the buttercup family and one of the first and most familiar spring flowers. The greater celandine contains violent poisons and only the homoeopathic preparations should be taken internally and according to medical advice. Take care too when using the juice externally to avoid letting it touch healthy skin when applying it to eczema etc. as it can itself produce sores. See my note in Part I under Dartres: Sundry methods.)

PREPARATION NO. 54A

Infusion of Greater Celandine

Put in a receptacle two tablespoonfuls of chopped fresh greater celandine leaves. Pour on a litre of boiling water. Stir, cover and leave to infuse for a quarter of an hour. Strain.

PREPARATION NO. 55

Cabbage Leaf Dressing *(Brassica oleracea)*

Principal indications: arteritis; renal colic; biliousness; sprains; carbuncles; haemorrhoids (piles); neuralgia; prostatitis; rheumatism

First wash and dry carefully the cabbage leaves to be used for a poultice. Remove the raised central rib and crush each leaf one by one with a rolling pin or bottle. Lay several leaves on top of one another over the affected area and cover with a woollen cloth held in place by a crêpe bandage which should not be too tight. The poultice should be kept unmoved for a few hours and then renewed. However, if the pain becomes unbearable the treatment should be allowed to lapse for a while. If a very tender wound is being treated the small ribs of the leaves should be removed as well as the central one and the leaves should be left to macerate in olive oil before use.

One can also cut strips from between the ribs or veins of the leaves and roll the pieces on themselves, as a cigar is rolled, to soften them. Place the portions of leaves on the wound as tiles are set on a roof, that is to say with the edge of one overlapping the other before applying a bandage to hold them in place.

PREPARATION NO. 56

Cabbage Poultice

Put in a saucepan three cabbage leaves, cut into small pieces with two finely-chopped onions. Add two handfuls of bran and mix with enough water to make a fairly liquid mash. Bring slowly to the boil, stirring constantly, and leave to cook until all the water has evaporated.

When it has cooled slightly, the preparation is laid on a fine cloth the edges of which are then folded over to make a poultice that should be somewhat larger than the affected area and of about two centimetres in thickness. Care must be taken not to apply the poultice too hot. Cover with a woollen cloth and hold in place with a bandage for about two hours.

PREPARATION NO. 57

Decoction of Oak Leaves *(Quercus robur)*

Principal indication: leucorrhoea ('whites')

Mix together equal quantities of oak leaves, eucalpytus leaves and white deadnettle leaves (the last not to be confused with stinging nettles) which should have been crumpled and broken to facilitate mixing. Put in a saucepan two tablespoonfuls of the leaves to a litre of cold water. Cover, bring slowly to the boil and leave to boil for five minutes before straining.

PREPARATION NO. 58

Decoction of Oak Bark

Principal indications: tonsilitis; diarrhoea; eczema; chilblains; gingivitis; impetigo; leucorrhoea

If for use as washes, gargles, enemas, douches – proceed in the following way: put in a saucepan six tablespoonfuls of crushed oak bark to a litre of cold water. Cover, bring slowly to the boil and leave to boil for ten minutes before straining.

If the decoction is intended as a beverage use four tablespoonfuls of oak bark fragments to a litre of cold water.

This decoction should not be prepared in an iron saucepan.

PREPARATION NO. 59

Oak Bark Wine

Principal indication: tonsilitis

Put in a litre bottle eight tablespoonfuls of crushed oak bark, fill with red wine and cork. Leave to macerate, shaking the bottle once a day for a week after which strain and decant into another bottle for storing.

PREPARATION NO. 60

Decoction of Oak Bark and Comfrey *(Quercus robur, Symphytum officinalis)*

Principal indication: too heavy periods

Put in a saucepan two tablespoonfuls of oak bark fragments and two tablespoonfuls of comfrey to a litre of cold water. Cover and bring to the boil slowly, boil for ten minutes and strain.

PREPARATION NO. 61

Decoction of Couchgrass *(Triticum repens)*

Principal indication: menopausal disorders

Put in a saucepan one tablespoonful of small pieces of couchgrass root to a litre of cold water. Cover and bring slowly to the boil. Leave on the boil for five minutes and strain.

PREPARATION NO. 62

Clematis Alcohol *(Clematis vitalba)*

Principal indications: arthritis; cellulite; neuritis; sciatica

(Translator's note: popular medicine does not specify whether wild or cultivated clematis is used but it is almost certainly only the wild plant that is intended. Our only native plant is *Clematis vitalba* and I have referred to it in this book as 'clematis' to avoid confusion that might arise from using one of its common English names: Traveller's Joy, Old Man's Beard, Virgin's Bower, etc.)

Put in a bottle 100 g of chopped fresh clematis leaves. Pour on half a litre of 70°alcohol. Leave to macerate, shaking the bottle once a day for a week. Then strain and bottle.

PREPARATION NO. 62A

Infusion of Clematis

Fresh clematis leaves are essential for this preparation. Put in a receptacle one tablespoonful of chopped clematis leaves. Pour on a litre of boiling water, stir well and leave to infuse for ten minutes. Strain.

PREPARATION NO. 63

Infusion of Quince Leaves *(Pyrus cydonia)*

Principal indications: insomnia; nervousness; coughing

Freshly-gathered quince leaves are needed for this preparation.

Put in a receptacle about ten chopped quince leaves. Pour on a litre of boiling water. Stir well, cover the receptacle and leave to infuse for ten minutes. Strain. Add to each cup half a coffee-spoonful of orange flower decoction.

PREPARATION NO. 64

Quince Wine

Principal indication: gingivitis

Dice a small unpeeled quince, put it in a bottle, fill up the bottle with white wine. Cork and leave to macerate for one week, shaking the bottle once a day. Strain. Decant into another bottle.

PREPARATION NO. 65

Infusion of Poppy *(Papaver rheas)*

Principal indications: tonsilitis; asthma; bronchitis; whooping cough; insomnia

Put in a saucepan a heaped tablespoonful of dried poppy petals. Pour on half a litre of boiling water, stir well and cover. Leave to infuse for ten minutes before straining.

This infusion should be well sweetened before being taken.

An infusion may also be prepared, particularly for cases of insomnia, with five whole poppy flowers which are left to infuse for ten minutes in a cup either of boiling water or of boiling milk.

PREPARATION NO. 66

Watercress Juice *(Nasturtium officinalis)*

Put through a mixer or sieve 100 g of fresh watercress and strain the juice which is then mixed with an equal quantity of vegetable broth. This preparation should be drunk cold.

PREPARATION NO. 67

Watercress Wine

Principal indications: anaemia; rickets; scurvy

Cut coarsely the leaves of a bunch of watercress and put them in a litre bottle. Fill with white wine. Cork and leave to macerate for two days, stirring from time to time. Then strain and bottle.

PREPARATION NO. 68

Infusion of Cumin *(Cummin cynenum)*

Principal indication: indigestion

Put in a receptacle three heaped coffeespoonfuls of cumin seeds. Pour on half a litre of boiling water, stir well, cover and leave to infuse for ten minutes before straining.

PREPARATION NO. 69

Decoction of Bittersweet *(Solanum dulcamara)*

Principal indications: Proteinuria; eczema

Chop into small pieces some bittersweet stems. Put three tablespoonfuls of them into a saucepan to a litre of cold water. Cover and leave to macerate for one hour. Bring slowly to the boil, boil for five minutes and strain. Sweeten the decoction with honey or sugar.

PREPARATION NO. 70

Infusion of Bittersweet or Woody Nightshade *(Solanum dulcamara)*

Principal indications: eczema; herpes; pleurisy; pneumonia; psoriasis

Put in a receptacle 100 g of chopped dried bittersweet. Pour on a litre and a half of boiling water, stir well and cover. Leave to infuse for six hours before straining. Before drinking the infusion sweeten it with honey or sugar.

PREPARATION NO. 71

Bittersweet Lotion

Principal indications: dartres; eczema; haemorrhoids; shingles; pruritis; psoriasis

Put in a saucepan 200 g of chopped stems of bittersweet to a litre of water. Either fresh of dried plants may be used but if fresh twigs are used add a small quantity of leaves. Cover and leave to macerate for six hours before bringing to the boil. Boil for five minutes before straining. Heat the lotion slightly before use.

PREPARATION NO. 72

Decoction of Dog Rose Hips *(Rosa canina)*

Principal indications: anxiety; insomnia; nausea; retention of urine; palpitation

Both fresh and dried dog rose hips can be used in this preparation. Put in a saucepan 50 g of dog rose hips that have been cut into two or three pieces to a litre of cold water. Cover, leave to macerate for three hours and then bring slowly to the boil. Boil for five minutes, macerate again for fifteen minutes, filter.

PREPARATION NO. 73

Liqueur of Dog Rose Hips

Principal indications: rickets; scurvy

Either fresh or dried hips may be used. Mix thoroughly in a large glass jar, such as a preserving jar, one kilo of dog rose hips cut into two or three pieces and 250 g of crystallized sugar. Pour on a litre and a half of *eau de vie,* cork and leave to macerate for three weeks, shaking the mixture once or twice a day. Strain and store in a bottle.

PREPARATION NO. 74

Dog Rose Hip Wine

Principal indications: dysentery; diarrhoea

As with the preceding preparations either dried or fresh hips may be used. Put in a bottle 50 g of dog rose hips cut into two or three pieces, fill with a good red wine, cork and leave to macerate for three days, shaking the bottle from time to time. Filter and add 200 g of sugar to the preparation.

PREPARATION NO. 75

Decoction of Barberries *(Berberis vulgaris)*

Principal indication: menopausal disorders

Use a mortar to crush 100 g of barberries, i.e. the fruit of the barberry shrub. Put them in a saucepan with a litre of cold water, cover and leave to soak for two hours. Bring slowly to the boil, boil for no more than a minute and wait until the decoction is tepid before straining it.

PREPARATION NO. 76

Decoction of Barberry Bark

Principal indication: toxicomania

Dried barberry root bark is needed for this preparation. Put in a saucepan five tablespoonfuls of the root bark to a litre of water. Cover and leave to soak for fifteen minutes. Bring slowly to the boil, boil for a few seconds and strain immediately.

PREPARATION NO. 77

Infusion of Eucalyptus *(Eucalyptus globulus)*

Principal indications: fever; cough

Put in a receptacle two tablespoonfuls of eucalyptus leaves cut into small pieces. Pour on a litre of boiling water, stir well, cover and leave to infuse for ten minutes before straining.

PREPARATION NO. 78

Decoction of Eucalyptus

Principal indications: bronchial disorders; influenza

Put in a saucepan three tablespoonfuls of chopped eucalyptus leaves to a litre of cold water. Cover, bring to the boil, boil for one minute. Leave to infuse for ten minutes before straining.

PREPARATION NO. 79

Eucalyptus Inhalation

Principal indications: bronchial disorders; influenza

Toss into a litre of boiling water a heaped tablespoonful of eucalyuptus leaves cut into small pieces. Boil for a few seconds, cover and leave to infuse for five minutes before inhaling.

PREPARATION NO. 80

Infusion of Fennel *(Foeniculum vulgare)*

Principal indications: asthma; whooping cough

Put in a saucepan a tablespoonful of fennel seeds. Pour on a litre of boiling water, stir for a while. Cover and leave to infuse for five minutes before straining. If seeds are not available, roots can be used instead in the proportions of three tablespoonfuls of finely-chopped fennel roots to a litre of water.

PREPARATION NO. 81

Decoction of Strawberry Roots *(Fragaria vesca)*

Principal indications: diarrhoea, kidney disorders

Either fresh or dried strawberry roots may be used for this preparation. Cut the roots into small pieces and put them into a saucepan, three tablespoonfuls to a litre of cold water. Cover and bring slowly to the boil. Leave to boil for ten minutes before straining.

PREPARATION NO. 82

Infusion of Strawberry Leaves

Principal indications: menstrual disorders

Put in a receptacle three tablespoonfuls of strawberry leaves cut into small pieces. Pour on a litre of boiling water, stir for a while, cover and leave to infuse for five minutes. Strain.

PREPARATION NO. 83

Decoction of Ash Leaves *(Fraxinus excelsior)*

Principal indications: facial neuralgia; rheumatism; slimming

Only dried leaves should be used for this preparation. Put in a saucepan three tablespoonfuls of chopped ash leaves to a litre of water. Cover, bring slowly to the boil, leave to boil for a quarter of an hour and strain. This infusion should be only slightly sweetened.

PREPARATION NO. 84

Infusion of Broom *(Sarothamnus scoparius* or *Cytisus scoparius)*

Principal indications: proteinuria; heart disorders; billousness; dropsy; nephritis; renal disorders

Put in a receptacle three tablespoonfuls of broom flowers. Pour on a litre of boiling water and stir for a while. Cover and leave to infuse for ten minutes before straining.

PREPARATION NO. 85

Decoction of Gentian *(Gentiana lutea)*

Principal indication: debility

Only dried roots of yellow gentian are used in this preparation. Put in a saucepan two tablespoonfuls of gentian roots cut into small pieces to a litre of cold water. Cover, bring slowly to the boil, leave boiling for ten minutes and strain.

PREPARATION NO. 86

Maceration of Gentian

Only dried roots, cut into small pieces, are used. Put in a saucepan one coffeespoonful of pieces of root to a cupful of cold water. Bring slowly to the boil, boil for ten minutes, leave to macerate through the night and strain only the following morning.

PREPARATION NO. 87

Mistletoe Wine *(Viscum album)*

Principal indications: arteriosclerosis; haemoptysis (spitting of blood)

Fresh leaves of mistletoe, cut into two or three pieces, are used for this preparation. Put in a litre bottle four tablespoonfuls of mistletoe leaves and fill with white wine. Cork and leave to macerate for a week, shaking the bottle once a day. Strain.

PREPARATION NO. 88

Decoction of Roots of Marsh Mallow *(Althaea officinalis)*

Principal indications: foot blisters; enemas for constipation and bowel inflammation

For an enema proceed in the following way: put in a saucepan three tablespoonfuls of segments of marsh mallow root to a litre of cold water. Cover, bring slowly to the boil, boil for fifteen minutes and strain.

For the care of the feet use 100 g of root to two litres of cold water.

PREPARATION NO. 89

Infusion of Marsh Mallow

Principal indication: bronchitis

Put in a receptacle two tablespoonfuls of marsh mallow flowers and leaves. Pour on a litre of boiling water, stir well, cover and leave to infuse for ten minutes before straining.

PREPARATION NO. 90

Infusion of Witch Hazel *(Hamamelis virginica)*

Principal indication: varicose veins

Either the dried leaves or bark of witch hazel may be used. Whichever is employed it should be cut or broken into small pieces and two tablespoonfuls and a teaspoonful of witch hazel put into a receptacle. Pour on a litre of boiling water, mix by stirring well, cover and leave to infuse for ten minutes. Strain.

PREPARATION NO. 91

Infusion of Bean Pods *(Phaseolus vulgaris)*

Principal indications: proteinuria; diabetes

The pods used in this preparation are those of the French, dwarf or runner bean and either dried or fresh pods may be used. If the pods are fresh, proceed in the following way: cut in small pieces two handfuls of bean pods. Put them in a saucepan with a litre of cold water. Cover, bring slowly to the boil, boil for two minutes and leave to macerate during the night, straining off the liquid next morning.

With dried pods, proceed as follows: cut a handful of pods into small pieces. Put them in a receptacle and pour on half a litre of boiling water. Stir, cover and leave to infuse for five minutes before straining.

PREPARATION NO. 92

Decoction of Herbs *(Rumex acetosa, Lactuca sativa, Allium porrum, Anthriscus cerefolium)*

Cut in small pieces 40 g of sorrel, 30 g of lettuce, 30 g of leeks and 20 g of chervil. Put the herbs in a saucepan to a litre and a half of cold water, bring slowly to the boil, boil for a quarter of an hour and strain.

PREPARATION NO. 93

Decoction of Lettuce Leaves *(Lactuca sativa)*

Principal indications: acne; constipation; insomnia; neuralgia; palpitations

To prepare this decoction choose the firmest lettuce you can find and preferably one that has started to 'bolt' or run to seed. Shred a few leaves of the lettuce and put six heaped tablespoonfuls to a litre of cold water. Cover, bring slowly to the boil, boil for quarter of an hour and strain.

PREPARATION NO. 94

Infusion of Lavender for external use *(Lavandula spica)*

Principal indications: acne; sores

Put in a receptacle three tablespoonfuls of lavender flowers. Pour on a litre of boiling water, mix by stirring well, cover and leave to infuse for twenty minutes. Strain. *(Translator's note:* the flowering tips of lavender only should be gathered for use in these preparations, picked before they have come to full bloom and dried in the shade.)

PREPARATION NO. 94A

Infusion of Lavender Flowers

Principal indications: asthma; whooping cough; nervous troubles

Put in a receptacle one tablespoonful of flowers. Pour on a litre of boiling water. Cover and leave to infuse for ten minutes and strain.

PREPARATION NO. 95

Infusion of Lavender Leaves

Principal indication: blotchiness of the face

Put in a receptacle two tablespoonfuls of leaves or sprigs of lavender. Pour on a litre of boiling water. Stir for a short while, cover and leave to infuse for six minutes before straining.

PREPARATION NO. 96

Oil of Lavender

Principal indication: eczema

Fresh lavender, chopped into small pieces, is used. First boil some water in a saucepan. In a small saucepan mix five tablespoonfuls of lavender flowers with half a litre of olive oil. Cook in a *bain marie* for two hours, i.e. put the small saucepan inside the larger one containing the water. Leave to macerate through the night and next morning filter through a fine cloth and then bottle.

PREPARATION NO. 97

Oil of Lily *(Lilium candidum)*

Principal indication: earache

Put in a receptacle 100 g of fresh Madonna lily petals to a quarter of a litre of olive oil. Cover and leave to macerate for a week stirring once daily. Transfer the preparation to a *bain marie* and simmer for three hours. Leave to macerate for three days and then filter through a fine cloth and store in a bottle.

PREPARATION NO. 98

Infusion of Bird's-Foot Trefoil *(Lotus corniculatus)*

Principal indication: anxiety

Put in a receptacle four tablespoonfuls of sprigs of flowering bird's-foot trefoil. Pour on a litre of boiling water. Stir well with a spoon, cover and leave to infuse for ten minutes and strain.

PREPARATION NO. 99

Infusion of Sweet Marjoram *(Origanum majorana)*

Principal indication: colds

Cut in small pieces some flowers and leaves of sweet marjoram. Place in a saucepan five tablespoonfuls of the prepared herb to a litre of boiling water. Stir the preparation, cover and leave to infuse for ten minutes before straining.

PREPARATION NO. 100

Decoction of Horse Chestnut *(Aesculus hippocastanum)*

Principal indication: haemorrhoids

Cut into small pieces the dried outer covering of the fruit (i.e. the spiky shells of the horse chestnuts or 'conkers' – *Translator's note)*. Put three tablespoonfuls to a litre of water. Cover, bring slowly to the boil, boil for ten minutes and strain.

PREPARATION NO. 101

Decoction of Horse Chestnut for external use

Principal indication: haemorrhoids

Crush coarsely some horse chestnut shells (see note above). Put in a saucepan ten tablespoonfuls to two litres of water. Cover, bring slowly to the boil, boil for a quarter of an hour and leave to infuse for five minutes before straining.

PREPARATION NO. 102

Decoction of Mallow and White Deadnettle *(Malva sylvestris, Lamium album)*

Principal indication: aphthas (small mouth ulcers)

Cut up some mallow flowers and leaves and some white deadnettle flowers and leaves (remember not to confuse with the stinging nettle or red deadnettle). Put in a saucepan one tablespoonful and one teaspoonful of mallow and the same quantity of white deadnettle to a litre of cold water. Cover, bring slowly to the boil, boil for five minutes and strain.

PREPARATION NO. 103

Infusion of Melilot *(Melilotus officinalis)*

Principal indication: insomnia

Cut in small pieces some dried melilot (the whole plant can be used). Put in a receptacle two tablespoonfuls of the chopped plant to a litre of water. Stir well, cover and leave to infuse for ten minutes before straining.

PREPARATION NO. 104

Infusion of Balm *(Melissa officinalis)*

Principal indications: stomach cramp; indigestion; insomnia; headaches; vomiting in pregnancy; nervous disorders

Either balm twigs or flowers or a mixture of the two may be used in this preparation. Put in a receptacle five tablespoonfuls of balm. Pour on a litre of boiling water. Stir well, cover and leave to infuse for ten minutes. Strain.

PREPARATION NO. 105

Balm Wine

Principal indication: fatigue

Cut into pieces some balm leaves. Put in a litre bottle eight tablespoonfuls of leaves. Fill the bottle with a good white wine, cork and leave to macerate for two days before straining.

PREPARATION NO. 106

Infusion of Mint *(Mentha)*

Principal indications: colic; difficult digestion: headaches: palpitations

Use mint leaves or a mixture of leaves and flowers. Put in a receptacle a heaped tablespoonful of mint and pour on half a litre of boiling water. Stir well, cover and leave to infuse ten minutes before straining.

PREPARATION NO. 107

Mint Wine

Principal indication: excessively light periods

Put in a receptacle one teaspoonful of mint leaves, one teaspoonful of rosemary sprigs, one teaspoonful of sage leaves and one of mugwort together with two bottles of claret. Macerate for one week, stirring once a day. Then strain and bottle.

PREPARATION NO. 108

Mint Lotion

Principal indication: blackheads

Mix in a flask 120 g of alcohol of mint with 80 g of rose water. Add 5 g of soluble aspirin to the mixture.

PREPARATION NO. 109

Oil of St John's Wort *(Hypericum perforatum)*

Principal indications: burns; sores; stomach ulcers; varicose ulcers

This preparation requires fresh flowers of St John's wort. Put in a glass receptacle 500 g of the flowers to a litre of olive oil. Macerate for ten days, leaving the receptacle in the sun, stirring the flowers two or three times a day. One the eleventh day strain and bottle.

PREPARATION NO. 110

Infusion of St John's Wort and White Deadnettle

Principal indication: inflammation of the urethra

Put in a receptacle four tablespoonfuls of flowers of St John's wort with four tablespoonfuls of the flowering tips of white deadnettle. Pour on a litre of boiling water. Stir well, cover and leave to infuse for ten minutes. Strain.

PREPARATION NO. 111

Infusion of Lily-of-the-Valley *(Convallaria majalis)*

Principal indications: palpitations; nervous excitability

Mix lily-of-the-valley flowers and their leaves, cut into pieces. Pour on half a litre of boiling water. Stir well, cover and allow to infuse for ten minutes before straining.

PREPARATION NO. 112

Decoction of Bilberries and Bilberry Leaves *(Vaccinium myrtillus)*

Principal indications: diabetes; eczema; enteritis

Mix some bilberries with their leaves, having cut the latter into pieces. Put in a saucepan four tablespoonfuls of this mixture to a litre of cold water. Cover, bring slowly to the boil and hold on the boil for ten minutes then strain.

PREPARATION NO. 113

Decoction of Bilberries

Principal indications: haemorrhoids; intestinal infections

Dried bilberries are used in this preparation.

Put in a saucepan five tablespoonfuls of bilberries to a litre of cold water. If the decoction is to be used as a beverage proceed in the following way: cover the saucepan and bring slowly to the boil, boil for five minutes and allow to infuse for a quarter of an hour. Strain, squeezing the berries to extract all the liquid.

For external use (particularly haemorrhoids): bring to the boil and keep on the boil until the liquid has been reduced to half the original volume. Strain at once, pressing the fruit well.

PREPARATION NO. 114

Bilberry Syrup

Principal indications: aphthas (mouth ulcers); enteritis; gingivitis

Fresh bilberries are used for this preparation. Put in a saucepan 250 g of bilberries, 250 g of sugar and add a quarter of a litre of water. Bring slowly to the boil and simmer until the liquid is reduced to a syrupy consistency. To strain, press the berries through a sieve, and then bottle.

PREPARATION NO. 115

Infusion of Walnut Leaves *(Juglans regia)*

Principal indications: anaemia; diabetes; eczema; high blood pressure; psoriasis

Cut into small pieces some walnut tree leaves, either fresh or dried. Put in a receptacle two tablespoonfuls of the cut leaves and pour on a litre of boiling water. Stir well, cover and allow to infuse for ten minutes before straining.

If walnut leaves are not available use in their place the same amount of dried outer husks of walnuts, cut into pieces.

PREPARATION NO. 116

Onion Wine *(Allium cepa)*

Principal indications: cramp; bilious attacks; lumbago; lumbar pains

Mince finely a pound of onions. Put them in a receptacle and mix with 150 g of honey. Add little by little and stirring all the time a litre of white wine. Cover and leave to macerate, stirring three or four times a day, for two days. Filter and bottle.

PREPARATION NO. 117

Samaritan's Balm

Principal indications: animal bites; mouth ulcers

Whisk briskly in a saucepan equal amounts of a good red wine and olive oil. Bring slowly to the boil and leave on the boil until the wine has completely evaporated. Allow to cool a little before transferring to the receptacle in which it is to be stored. *(Translator's note:* named with accuracy as well as piety, this preparation was obviously inspired by Luke 10:33-34:

33 But a certain Samaritan, as he journeyed, came where he was: and when he saw him, he had compassion on him.

34 And went to him, and bound up his wounds, pouring in oil and wine, and set him on his own beast, and brought him to an inn, and took care of him.)

PREPARATION NO. 118

Infusion of Olive Leaves *(Olea europaea)*

Principal indication: high blood pressure

Cut into two or three pieces some leaves from an olive tree. Put the leaves into a receptacle, about one and half tablespoonfuls to half a litre of boiling water. Stir, cover and leave to infuse five minutes before straining.

PREPARATION NO. 119

Infusion of Orange Flowers and Leaves *(Citrus aurantium)*

Principal indications: bronchitis; colic; insomnia; hiccups; cough; nervous excitability

Orange blosson is used in the case of colic and the leaves of the orange tree for the other indications.

Put in a receptacle two tablespoonfuls of the herb and pour on a litre of boiling water. Stir well and cover. If flowers are used leave to infuse for ten minutes, and give leaves a fifteen-minute infusion, before straining.

If the infusion is taken for insomnia add just before drinking a teaspoonful of orange flower water.

PREPARATION NO. 120

Infusion of Lime (Linden) and Orange *(Tilia europaea and Citrus aurantium)*

Principal indication: nervous excitability

Put in a receptacle a level tablespoonful of lime (linden) with the same amount of orange flowers or leaves. Pour on half a litre of boiling water, stir, cover and leave to infuse for ten minutes before straining.

PREPARATION NO. 121

Decoction of Elm *(Ulmus campertris)*

Principal indications: dartres, leucorrhoea; psoriasis

Coarsely-crushed elm bark is generally used in this preparation but if none is obtainable use instead some chopped elm leaves. Put in a receptacle six tablespoonfuls of the herb to a litre of cold water. Cover, leave to soak for two hours and then bring slowly to the boil for three minutes. Allow to infuse for fifteen minutes before straining.

PREPARATION NO. 122

Elm Ointment

Principal indications: dartres; psoriasis

Use chopped dried elm bark for this preparation.

Mix in a saucepan five tablespoonfuls of the bark with 50 g of oil of almonds and 50 g of beeswax. Heat in a *bain marie* and bring the mixture to the boil three times and only for a second each time. Filter immediately through a fine cloth and store in a jar.

PREPARATION NO. 123

Decoction of Stinging Nettles *(Urtica dioica)*

Principal indications: anaemia; leucorrhoea; heavy periods; rheumatism; psoriasis

For this preparation the dried stalks and leaves of stinging nettles are cut into small pieces before use.

Put in a saucepan three tablespoonfuls of the herb to half a litre of cold water. Cover, bring slowly to the boil, boil for five minutes and allow to infuse for ten minutes before straining.

PREPARATION NO. 124

Infusion of White Deadnettle *(Lamium album)*

Principal indication: metritis (inflammation of the uterus)

Put in a receptacle six tablespoonfuls of the flowering tips of white deadnettle and pour on a litre of boiling water. Stir well, cover and leave to infuse for ten minutes before straining.

PREPARATION NO. 125

Infusion of Pellitory-of-the-Wall *(Parietaria officinalis)*

Principal indications: diarrhoea; disorders of the urinary tract

Cut into pieces some leaves and flowering tips of pellitory-of-the-wall. Place three tablespoonfuls in a receptacle and pour on half a litre of boiling water. Stir, cover and allow to infuse for ten minutes before straining.

PREPARATION NO. 126

Decoction of Parsley *(Apium petroselinum)*

Principal indications: circulation disorders; backache; retention of urine; irregular periods

In this preparation seeds, dried roots or fresh leaves and stalks of parsley may be used.

If seeds or roots are used proceed in the following manner: put in a saucepan one tablespoonful of seeds or five tablespoonfuls of chopped roots to a litre of cold water. Cover, bring slowly to the boil, boil for a few seconds and leave to infuse for twenty minutes before straining.

If fresh parsley is used, chop the leaves and stems. Put in a receptacle two tablespoonfuls of chopped parsley. Pour on half a litre of boiling water. Stir, cover and leave to infuse for ten minutes before straining.

PREPARATION NO. 127

Infusion of Periwinkle *(Vinca minor)*

Principal indications: tonsilitis; sore throat

Use either the leaves or the dried flowers of periwinkle. If the preparation is made with leaves, put in a saucepan six tablespoonfuls of leaves that have been cut into pieces to a litre of cold water. Cover and bring slowly to the boil, boil for ten minutes and strain.

If using dried flowers only two tablespoonfuls are needed. Pour on a litre of boiling water, stir well, cover and allow to infuse for ten minutes before straining.

PREPARATION NO. 128

Decoction of Dandelion *(Taraxacum officinalis)*

Principal indications: calculia (stones); skin diseases

Either dandelion roots or chopped fresh dandelion leaves may be used but a mixture of the two is preferable.

Put in a receptacle six tablespoonfuls of the herb to a litre of cold water. Cover, bring slowly to the boil and allow to boil ten minutes before straining.

PREPARATION NO. 129

Infusion of Dandelion

Principal indication: biliousness

Use roots or leaves as for preparation No. 128.

Put in a receptacle five tablespoonfuls of the herb. Pour on a litre of boiling water, stir well, cover and allow to infuse for ten minutes before straining.

PREPARATION NO. 130

Decoction of Field Horsetail *(Equisetum arvense)*

Principal indications: inflammation of the urinary tract; incontinence of urine; haemorrhages; heavy periods
Use the dried herb, cut into small pieces.

Put in a saucepan five tablespoonfuls of herb to a litre of cold water. Cover and leave to macerate for two hours. Bring slowly to the boil, boil for ten minutes and strain.

PREPARATION NO. 131

Infusion of Field Horsetail

Principal indication: decalcification
Use all parts of the herb, dried and cut into small pieces. Put in a receptacle two tablespoonfuls of the herb and pour on half a litre of boiling water. Stir well, cover and allow to infuse for ten minutes before straining.

PREPARATION NO. 132

Tincture of Field Horsetail

Principal indication: excessive perspiration of the feet
Drop into a bottle 200 g of field horsetail that has been cut into small pieces. Pour on 200 g of 90° alcohol. Cork and leave to macerate for one week, shaking the bottle two or three times a day. Strain at the end of the seven days.

PREPARATION NO. 133

Decoction of Horseradish Root *(Cochlearia armorica* or *Raphanus rusticanus)*

Principal indications: asthenia (debility); gout
Use fresh horseradish root, cut into small pieces.

Put in a saucepan two tablespoonfuls of horseradish to a litre of cold water. Cover, bring slowly to the boil, boil for five minutes before straining.

PREPARATION NO. 134

Decoction of Liquorice *(Glycyrrhiza glabra)*

Principal indications: tonsilitis; bronchitis; constipation; cystitis; stomach cramps; colds
Use the root of liquorice, cut into small pieces.

Put in a saucepan five tablespoonfuls of liquorice to a litre of cold water. Cover, bring slowly to the boil, boil for five minutes and leave to macerate for twelve hours before straining.

PREPARATION NO. 135

Infusion of Liquorice

Principal indication: conjunctivitis

Use the root of liquorice, cut into small pieces.

Put in a receptacle seven tablespoonfuls of liquorice root. Pour on a litre of boiling water, stir well, cover and leave to infuse for one hour before straining.

PREPARATION NO. 136

Maceration of Liquorice

Principal indications: constipation; irritation of the eyes

Use the stem of liquorice, cut into small pieces.

Put in a saucepan five tablespoonfuls of liquorice to a litre of cold water. Cover and leave to macerate for six hours. Bring slowly to the boil, boil for five minutes and allow to settle for six hours before straining.

PREPARATION NO. 137

Infusion of Meadowsweet *(Spiraea ulmaria)*

Principal indications: arthritis, rheumatism

For this preparation use either fresh of dried flowers mixed with a few leaves, if possible.

Put in a receptacle five tablespoonfuls of the herb. Bring a litre of water to the boil. Let it cool gradually and when cold pour it on the meadowsweet, stirring well. Cover, leave to infuse for ten minutes before straining.

PREPARATION NO. 138

Meadowsweet Wine

Principal indication: fever

For this preparation either fresh or dried flowers may be used. Put in a saucepan three tablespoonfuls of flowers to a litre of white wine. Bring slowly to the boil for ten minutes before straining.

Allow the wine to settle for twenty-four hours in a well-covered receptacle before bottling.

PREPARATION NO. 139

Infusion of Rhubarb *(Rheum officinalis)*

Principal indications: constipation; acidity; neurasthenia

Use dried rhubarb root cut into small pieces.

Put in a receptacle one tablespoonful and one coffeespoonful of rhubarb root. Pour on half a litre of boiling water. Stir well, cover and leave to infuse for a quarter of an hour before straining.

PREPARATION NO. 140

Infusion of Rosemary *(Roemarinus officinalis)*

Principal indications: asthma; whooping cough; insomnia

For this preparation use flowering sprigs of rosemary, cut in pieces.

Put in a receptacle four coffeespoonfuls of rosemary. Pour on a litre of boiling water. Stir well and leave to infuse for ten minutes before straining.

PREPARATION NO. 141

Rosemary Wine

Principal indications: stomach ache; painful periods

For this preparation use flowering sprigs of rosemary, cut in pieces.

Put in a litre bottle six tablespoonfuls of rosemary and fill the bottle with white wine. Cork and leave to macerate for two weeks, shaking the bottle once a day. Filter.

PREPARATION NO. 142

Decoction of Soapwort *(Saponaria officinalis)*

Principal indication: skin diseases

Use either soapwort root or flowers for this preparation.

If the root is being used put in a receptacle five tablespoonfuls to a litre of water: three tablespoonfuls if flowes are used. Put in a saucepan the herb with the water, cover and bring slowly to the boil. Boil for ten minutes before straining. It is important to strain at once because if allowed to stand the decoction could develop toxic properties.

PREPARATION NO. 143

Infusion of Soapwort

Principal indications: herpes; impetigo; shingles
Use either soapwort leaves or dried roots for this preparation.

The infusion can be drunk or can be applied as a lotion. In the first case put in a receptacle two tablespoonfuls of the herb and pour on a litre of boiling water. Stir well, cover and leave to infuse for five minutes before straining. In the second case, proceed in the same way but instead of two tablespoonfuls put five to a litre of boiling water.

PREPARATION NO. 144

Decoction of Sage *(Salvia officinalis)*

Principal indications: mouth ulcers; sore throat; thrush
Either leaves or flowering sprigs of sage may be used for this preparation and the herb can be fresh or dried.

Put in a saucepan five tablespoonfuls of the herb to a litre of cold water. Cover, bring slowly to the boil, boil for ten minutes and allow to infuse for another ten minutes before straining.

PREPARATION NO. 145

Infusion of Sage

Principal indications: swollen legs, stomach ache; tender gums; menopausal disorders; neurasthenia; painful periods; excessive sweating
Use flowers or flowering sprigs of sage, either fresh or dried.

Put in a receptacle two tablespoonfuls of the herb and pour on a litre of boiling water. Stir well, cover and leave to infuse for ten minutes. Strain. The infusion can also be prepared with milk: one tablespoonful to a litre of boiling milk. Leave to infuse for twelve minutes before straining.

PREPARATION NO. 146

Infusion of Sage for external use

Put in a receptacle three tablespoonfuls of flowers or leaves of sage. Pour on half a litre of boiling water and stir well. Leave to infuse for ten minutes and then strain.

PREPARATION NO. 147

Sage Wine

Principal indications: asthenia (debility); excessive sweating

Put in a litre bottle ten tablespoonfuls of sage leaves. Fill up the bottle with muscatel wine. Cork and leave to macerate for one week, shaking the bottle once a day. Filter and decant into a bottle.

PREPARATION NO. 148

Infusion of Willow *(Salix alba)*

Principal indication: neurasthenia

Use fresh leaves of willow. *(Translator's note:* the French original does not specify which of over 300 species of the family *Salicaceae* is used in this preparation but it can be reasonably assumed that the White Willow, *Salix alba,* widely used in remedies, is intended.) Cut into two or three pieces. Put in a receptacle one tablespoonful and one coffeespoonful of leaves and pour on half a litre of boiling water. Stir well, cover and leave to infuse for ten minutes before straining.

PREPARATION NO. 149

Decoction of Hedge Mustard *(Sisymbrium officinale)*

Principal indication: hoarseness

The common French name for hedge mustard is 'herbe aux chantres' or 'chorister's herb' since it is the specific for the vocal cords. The whole plant can be used, cut into small pieces.

Put in a saucepan three tablespoonfuls of hedge mustard to a litre of cold water. Cover, bring slowly to the boil, boil for ten minutes and strain.

PREPARATION NO. 150

Infusion of Marigold *(Calendula officinalis)*

Principal indications: chilblains; stomach ache; skin diseases

Use either leaves or flowers of marigold.

Put in a receptacle three tablespoonfuls of dried marigold. Pour on a litre of boiling water. Stir well, cover and leave to infuse for ten minutes and then strain. If fresh marigold is used, proceed in the same way but use only two tablespoonfuls of the plant instead of three.

PREPARATION NO. 151

Infusion of Elder *(Sambucus nigra)*

Principal indications: influenza; neuralgia; colds; measles

The flowers of elder are used for this preparation.

Put in a receptacle five tablespoonfuls of elder flowers. Pour on a litre of boiling water. Stir well, cover and leave to infuse for ten minutes before straining.

PREPARATION NO. 152

Elder Water

Principal indication: blackheads

Put in a receptacle two tablespoonfuls of elder flowers and one teaspoonful of senna (if senna is unobtainable add an extra tablespoonful of elder flowers). Pour on half a litre of boiling water. Stir well, cover and leave to infuse for a quarter of an hour before straining.

PREPARATION NO. 153

Infusion of Tansy *(Tanacetum vulgare)*

Principal indications: aerophagia; muscular cramp; sprains; haemorrhoids; indigestion; leucorrhoea, nervous disorders

For this preparation use the dried flowering sprigs of tansy cut into small pieces.

Put in a receptacle four tablespoonfuls of tansy. Pour on a litre of boiling water, cover and leave to infuse for ten minutes before straining.

PREPARATION NO. 154

Bath with Thyme *(Thymus vulgaris)*

Principal indications: debility; asthenia

Put in a large receptacle 500 g of thyme to four litres of cold water. Bring slowly to the boil, boil for five minutes, leave to infuse for a quarter of an hour, strain and add the preparation to the bathwater.

PREPARATION NO. 155

Decoction of Thyme

Principal indication: colds

Cut in small pieces a medium-sized sprig of thyme.

Put the pieces of thyme in a saucepan and pour on a cupful of boiling water. Bring back to the boil for a few seconds and then infuse for ten minutes before straining.

PREPARATION NO. 156

Infusion of Thyme

Principal indications: asthenia, influenza; neuralgia; rheumatoid arthritis; diseases of the respiratory tract

Cut into small pieces some sprigs of thyme.

Put in a receptacle two tablespoonfuls of thyme. Pour on a cupful of boiling water. Stir well, cover and leave to infuse for ten minutes. Strain.

PREPARATION NO. 157

Infusion of Lime (Linden) *(Tilia europaea)*

Principal indications: gout; headaches

Put in a receptacle one tablespoonful of lime flowers. Pour on half a litre of boiling water, stir well, cover and leave to infuse for ten minutes before straining.

PREPARATION NO. 158

Decoction of Lime

Principal indications: indigestion; insomnia; lumbago; headaches; rheumatism; circulatory disorders

Put in a saucepan five tablespoonfuls of lime flowers to a litre of cold water. Cover, bring slowly to the boil, boil for a quarter of an hour and strain.

PREPARATION NO. 159

Bath with Lime (Linden)

Principal indication: nervous excitability

Put in a large receptacle 500 g of lime flowers and pour on five litres of boiling water. Stir and mix well, cover and leave to infuse for a quarter of an hour. Strain and add the infusion to the bathwater.

PREPARATION NO. 160

Infusion of Valerian *(Valeriana officinalis)*

Principal indications: asthma, stitch; high blood pressure; insomnia; menopausal disorders; headaches; restless sleep

Use the root of valerian, dried and cut into small pieces.

Put in a receptacle six tablespoonfuls of valerian root. Boil a litre of water and as soon as it has cooled pour it on the valerian. Leave to soak during the night and filter it the following morning.

PREPARATION NO. 160A

Bath with Valerian

Use root of valerian, dried and chopped as finely as possible.

Put 200 g of root to two litres of cold water. Leave to macerate for about ten hours. Bring slowly to the boil and boil for about ten minutes, strain and then add the decoction to the bathwater.

PREPARATION NO. 161

Decoction of Veronica or Common Speedwell *(Veronica officinalis)*

Principal indications: aerophagia; biliousness; dartres; indigestion; gingivitis; sore throat; depression; sores

For this preparation use a mixture of dried leaves and flowers of veronica. *(Translator's note:* the French original does not specify which of the speedwells should be used of the dozen species that exist but, referring back to the Latin, it is obviously the Common speedwell, Veronica officinalis i.e. 'used medicinally'. To lessen likelihood of confusion with other speedwells I have used 'veronica' throughout the book.)

Put in a saucepan ten tablespoonfuls of veronica to a litre of cold water. Cover, bring slowly to the boil, boil for ten minutes, leave to infuse for a further ten minutes, then strain.

PREPARATION NO. 162

Infusion of Veronica

Principal indications; aerophagia; asthma; bronchitis; indigestion; migraine.

Use leaves of veronica that have been dried and lightly crushed.

Put in a receptacle ten tablespoonfuls of veronica. Pour on a litre of boiling water, stir well, cover and leave to infuse for twenty minutes before straining.

PREPARATION NO. 163

Verbena or Vervain Poultice *(Verbena officinalis)*

Principal indication: stitch

Use dried and crushed verbena leaves.

Put in a saucepan ten tablespoonfuls of verbena leaves to a decilitre of vinegar. Bring slowly to the boil and keep it boiling until a thick preparation is obtained which is then wrapped in gauze and applied to the aching side.

PREPARATION NO. 164

Decoction of Verbena

Principal indications: cellulite; colic; stitch; stomach ache; fatigue; fever; headache or migraine; facial neuralgia

Dried verbena leaves are used for this preparation.

Put five tablespoonfuls of verbena to a litre of cold water. Cover, leave to macerate for two hours then bring slowly to the boil. Allow to boil for thirty seconds then let it infuse for a quarter of an hour before straining.

PREPARATION NO. 165

Infusion of Verbena

Principal indications: stomach ache; headaches and migraine

The whole plant is used for this preparation, cut into small pieces.

Put in a receptacle a coffeespoonful of verbena. Pour on a cupful of boiling water. Stir well, cover, leave to infuse for ten minutes and then strain.

PREPARATION NO. 166

Decoction of Vine Leaves *(Vitis vinifera)*

Principal indications: cellulite; obesity; chilblains; haemorrhoids; blotchiness of the face; varicose veins

Use dried vine leaves, lightly crushed.

Put in a saucepan six tablespoonfuls of leaves to a litre of cold water. Cover, bring slowly to the boil, boil for five minutes and leave to infuse for a quarter of an hour before straining.

PREPARATION NO. 167

Decoction of Violets *(Viola odorata)*

Principal indications: tonsilitis; aphtas; bronchitis; whooping cough; cystitis; fever; gingivitis; influenza; migraine; skin diseases; colds; retention of urine

Dried violet flowers are used for this preparation.

Put in a saucepan five tablespoonfuls of violets to a litre of cold water. Cover, heat slowly and remove from the heat at the moment it comes to the boil. Leave to infuse for a quarter of an hour before straining.

Herbs used in the Preparations

Common English Name / Number of the preparation